Eat Yourself Younger ...Effortlessly

The easy way to slow aging, feel great, and look good.

By: Celia Westberry, M.S.

**Book cover and graphics by
Christian Weigand**

Praise for Celia Westberry and Eat Yourself Younger Effortlessly

"Eat Yourself Younger ... Effortlessly," delivers the promise to give you information to feel younger, look better, and live longer by using "body friendly foods." The knowledge is captured simply, clearly, and holistically. Recipes, and other directions can be easily followed, and the information shows Health Coach Celia Westberry's integrity and compelling competence. Delight your body and your spirit. Read, digest, and act on this wisdom, if you want to live a better life.

---Philip Guy Rochford, Success Coach and Author of Infinite Possibilities & The Executive Speaks.

Celia Westberry makes eating what your body wants tasty. Move over Dr. Perricone, Westberry's way is here! I love the recipes and menu plans, so much more effective than leaving us to figure out how to implement the right foods into our lives.

---Stephanie Bacak, Owner, Frontier Marketing International, LLC

This book should have happened a long time ago. It is good for the person who is busy and needs to depend on a reference for good, wholesome and tasteful food, without using a lot of effort and time.

---Pearl Smith, Attorney at law

If you follow the hints and directions given and eat from the recipes in this book, you will have a more satisfying, fulfilling and healthy life!

---Chef Mark Powers

I personally have had the opportunity to eat and enjoy many of Celia's dishes. She really knows how to combine food to be nutritious and taste wonderful,

---Cindy Burrows, Herbalist and Nutrition Consultant

Acknowledgements

This 2nd edition of "Eat Yourself Younger – Effortlessly" exist because of an insight I was given in a short conversation with T. Havr Eker about giving your best. He practices what he preaches, he gives and gives…; I hope to do the same!

To Ryan Newhouse - thanks for your keen eye and editing skills and for the fact that you loved reading about food. Working with Ryan is a delightful exercise in promptness and efficiency.

My deepest gratitude goes to Chris Weigand for his sense of generosity that is reveled in his gift of creativity. Your sensibility about what I wanted for the cover layout of this book is amazing. I am in awe and I hope everyone who sees this cover will be also.

To Tracy Colvill, thank you for your timely unsolicited attention. Giving me comments, critique and encouragement at the moment I needed it is true serendipity.

Thanks to my husband Larry who gave this book visual impact, masterminded the photography while reluctantly dealing with my whim and crazy manner of deciding what I wanted.

To Treasure Gains Oines for the original layout of this book and for her selfless friendship, a heart-felt thank you. Treasure you really are a gem.

My gratitude goes to Mark Victor Hansen for nurturing authors. His Mega Book seminars revealed to me the magnitude of my challenge and how to direct my mission; which is to use books to initiate the change I want to see in the world.

DEDICATION

This book is dedicated to the memory of my sweet Aunt Eva who took me from fear and frustration to daring and pleasure in her lessons about food and cooking.

And to my cousin Ewart Roett who urged me to write down my recipes.

Forward

In retrospect, the seeds of Eat Yourself Younger Effortlessly were born when I was about 5 years old. My father died. I grieved! I also learned the word, diabetes. I grew up determined to find out about this disease that plucked my father away in a coma, - a here today, gone tomorrow episode. Because of my quest, I became painfully aware that certain foods can sustain life, as well as destroy. Take a look at sugar, the favorite comfort food to crave, it is entirely necessary for brain energy, but an excess in your blood is called diabetes and can kill.

Fortunately, in pursuit of my purpose I met some wonderful people, with the generosity of spirit ready to help me achieve my goals. It started when as an undergraduate, Dr. Alberta Seaton; my first mentor helped me to get a National Science Foundation Summer Grant. This experience left me in complete awe of the mysteries of animal cells and their DNA.

I then had the good fortune to be the graduate student of Dr. S. Venketeswaran.   As a botanist expert in cell biology, he helped to me gain insights into the power and potency of plant cells. Also, there was Dr. David Mumford who had the courage to let me freely use his state of the art cell biology lab at Baylor College of Medicine, Houston to do my graduate research, even though I was enrolled at the University of Houston.
As I got more involved with scientific research, the one thing that left a big impression with me was the need for frequency of feeding of cells, in order to sustain optimum cell life. Another eye opener was the action of the required chemicals in their food that worked with absolute synergy, to maintain healthy cell cultures.

But let's not complicate feeding. The universal plan is simple. Nature has been perfecting food with the chemical synergy of compounds such as antioxidants and vitamins for billions and billons of years, just for our choosing. Fresh food comes with this kind natural combination of chemical materials that we manage to mimic in scientific research. We just have to make wise choices from a wide array of fresh food.

I taught cell and molecular biology for 10 years, before the light bulb went of in my head that the best way to keep a human body from premature aging, is to give body cells what is absolutely necessary for optimum health. This happens through eating. With this epiphany, I explored the idea of 'eating younger', and how each meal contributes to optimum health. So far, with this idea I have already lived 2 decades longer than my father and have not succumbed to my genetic link to diabetes, or any other aging illness for that matter...

Eat Yourself Younger Effortlessly can be the breakthrough you are seeking if you are at the crossroads of health... It is designed   to help you make natural food choices. My hope is that you will open this book and use it to eat to your colon, brain and heart's content.

The Ideas and concepts in Eat Yourself Younger Effortlessly will get you centered on happy, healthy aging. This is your bridge from fad nutrition, crazy unhealthy beliefs, yo–yo dieting and so-so eating habits, to simple but powerful eating choices. You now have the tools. They are the well designed menus and recipes that pay attention to glycemic load, portion size, and full strength chemical energy in food. And they are delicious.

These natural gifts of nature will keep you free of lifestyle symptoms, caused by poor food choices, which eventually lead to unwieldy illnesses of aging. Can you imagine not having to fight cancer, because you eat foods that constantly support your immune system, nature's gift for fighting disease? You now have more possibilities for success and joy, using the body friendly foods in this book.

My wish for you is that Eat Yourself Younger Effortlessly will bring passion and purpose to your eating. I envision use of this book taking you to a higher level of sustenance, where human

energy is created from fresh food. With this bounty you have the power to slow your aging, feel great and look good.

Introduction – Anti-aging Cuisine - EAT YOURSELF YOUNGER...EFFORTLESSLY

I first made a connection about the wonders of food when I was about 7 years old. I was reading a book about fruit when I discovered that the seed in an apple was actually a tree just waiting for someone to plant it. It was such a wonder: that little seed and that big tree, with its potency to bear even more fruit. It was too miraculous. Growing up in the Tropics, I would think of the mysterious biblical Adam and Eve's first bite, and I would long to pick an apple dangling from a tree. What I did do, though, was make the connection with how small things in food can be very powerful. Now it is easy for me to accept the wisdom behind the saying, "an apple a day keeps the doctor away." What else is in that apple? The information is growing. For instance, there is a soluble fiber called pectin that give us necessary bulk, helps us feel full, and plays a part in lowering high levels of cholesterol. Also, to add to the mystery, the apple's seed should not be eaten because it contains cyanide, which is a deadly poison. One or two seeds would not hurt but an overload can kill. This lets me know that portion size is important. What other complexities does this one fruit have to offer? Could this fruit contain a wonder drug waiting to take the place of the fountain of youth? One major possibility is that food can play a significant role in delaying the inevitability of aging.

It is no secret that what we choose to put in our mouths has a tremendous effect on how we look and feel. Have you noticed how a baby can thrive on his mother's milk until he is a walking, talking toddler? After which, he has to eat a wider variety of food to help him mature into a budding teenager. At this junction in his life, he uses up most of this food energy in growing and developing various organ systems. When all this growth and development settles down, we are left with having to maintain our body systems. Now we need a change in diet that helps to resist decline at an early age. But by this time we have ingrained habits, a sweet-tooth and a propensity to live on certain favorite foods, like pepperoni pizza, or French-fries and a burger, foods that are familiar to the culture where we grew up. This can serve us through adolescence, but as we continue to mature, we might see changes in our weight and health that let us know we need a different kind of nutritional support; one that will support our youthfulness, as nature changes the process of building into one of maintaining. The premise is to choose foods that give all the benefits needed to prolong your youth. This is a chance to open your awareness toward understanding that every opportunity to eat is a chance to give yourself a piece of nature that can help your body resist aging. The fringe benefit is that you will also maintain your health well into maturity. One of the best compliments I've received was from a young college student who said that I was the fittest-looking mature woman she has seen in our area. I really value that because one of my goals as I grow older is to stay well and fit. I have been thinking about aging for the past decade, not because I am afraid of sagging skin or wrinkles, but because sometimes symptoms of aging show up as annoying aches, pains and various indications of ill health, such as heart problems. The recipes in this book contain food that has many of the vitamins and minerals in supplements that are recommended to keep us youthful and stop annoying symptoms of aging. The idea here is to use natural food to support maturing body organ systems and to avoid these aging symptoms. For instance, there are recipes that mention supporting your immune system instead of merely helping with a common cold or arthritic pains. I am not a trained chef, but my background as a cellular biologist helps me to see food at the miraculous chemical and cellular level, where all life starts, develops and is maintained. I have cooked for a family for three decades and have experimented and proven how food can heal, especially when dealing with diseases like diabetes, hypoglycemia and gout that respond to changes in food plans. What I can do in my kitchen, you can also do.

This book helps you to sustain yourself with quality food and do it in a way that is harmonious with the way we live now. We live in a time when it is just as easy to grab a prepared fast-food meal, as it is to get the freshest, most invigorating food and prepare it at home. At home we have all the modern conveniences that make food preparation effortless and fast. It's your choice. The recipes and information presented here give you choices that will help you keep your vigor and vitality for as long as you please.

This book has recipes and hints that focus on the foods that maintain youthfulness, if eaten regularly. And the extra special gift is that your internal organ systems will remain in tiptop shape, which translates to better health and less syndromes and symptoms of aging.

The recipes serve one or two persons so that it is easy to pay attention to portion size. Because no matter how good a food is for you, more is not better. When I was working as a research scientist, I was responsible for growing human cells for experiments. Growth demands feeding and these cells had to be fed with certain regularity. One of my main jobs was to make up the formula or recipe. Once the right recipe for growth was determined, the cells flourished and the cell culture looked good and grew well. If I added too much or too little of a substance, perhaps simply because I was low on an ingredient and thought I could compensate by adding more of another, it really sent my cells into a tizzy. They looked terrible, curled up their membranes and became stressed. Some cells actually aged before their time and died. All of that occurred because of not meeting a simple ingredient quantity parameter. From this I now know that portion size and having the right ingredients are fundamentally important. These recipes are neither low-fat, high-protein, or overloaded with carbohydrates. The idea here was to strive for a supportive balance. Another important aspect is the rhythm of feeding. Those cells did not like changes in their feeding times. They had to be fed often and on time. The recipes in this book were chosen to meet the needs of people who desire to avoid nutritional stress and keep cells young. The idea is to give continued support to the tissues and organ systems that are involved in helping you avoid premature aging.

For me, cooking effortlessly is to bring into full play the modern conveniences of kitchen appliances and gadgets. I use modern conveniences, like cooking with a microwave, food processors, high-speed blenders and even a not-so-modern invention, the pressure cooker. It is a good idea to have as many state of the art accessories as you can afford. Your friends and family will notice that you are on this cooking quest and will be relieved to know that you would love to receive gifts of knives, peelers, tongs, whisks, fancy strainers and bowls.

All of these things help make your time in the kitchen more enjoyable. I have found that it is always easier to succeed when you have the precise instruments at hand. Then, all you will need is a great big bout of enthusiasm and self-love. Also, remember to pencil in some time in your calendar to cook.

I believe that getting very involved in preparing your own food is nurturing, and spiritually uplifting. It keeps you in the survival game of hunting and gathering. In a modern harmonious way, it is fun and challenging to find and prepare the freshest foods in season from grocery stores, farmers markets or even your own garden.

If you have a passion for cooking with a variety of fresh foods and are seeking to get more substance from your foods, then using this book will add purpose to your cooking and give you more options. I did not include the actual measurements of grams of fat, proteins or sugar. In most of the recipes, the fat used is good vegetable fat. Sugar and fiber is mostly naturally-occurring in the foods, and the protein content is 3 or 4 ounces per serving. The recipes give you a healthy balance.

There are chapters for breakfast, lunch, dinner and snacks so that you can always have a choice of foods and can bypass any kind of deprivation. Once you make a choice, you can easily develop a menu for the coming week from examples given. This helps to create a new, better habit of cooking and eating.

You are going to love this book:

- **If you want to cook a variety of foods that are deliciously powerful as well as balancing, and help you to look good as you age.**
- **If you want more options, more knowledge and more experience with different kinds of beneficial food.**
- **If you are seeking more confidence in making new choices with meals.**
- **If you have been battling food cravings, and illness associated with aging and food. You will notice that our menus are balanced for sugar and starches, and our recipes serve one or two persons, so it is easy not to overload on any one food. Therefore, you will not gain weight, and you might even lose some inches in desirable places, like your mid-riff.**
- **If you are concerned about degenerative diseases caused by imbalances in nutrition, and want to stay well as you mature.**
- **If you just want more energy and you are at that stage in life where it's necessary to continuously multi-task.**

Most of all, food should nurture your soul as well as your body, so cook from this book if you want to delight your spirit.

My wish is that you will find these recipes deliciously satisfying and that the process of cooking will take your ideas of nurturing yourself to a higher, more beneficial level.

The Effortless Plan

Nothing worthwhile comes from a single effort. First is deliberate effort, focused on timing and attention. Then there is a certain, practiced rhythm, until the mind and body picks it up at the unconscious level, like knowing the way to work without thinking. Somehow you get there everyday, knowing all the stops and bumps along the way, and you do it with competence, never missing a turn. Somehow you and your vehicle get there without much thought. But things were not always so! First you had to learn to drive, and then pick the car that was suitable for you. You had to plan and learn directions, and make some choices about the journey. Well, cooking is like that. First you get the tools, then the ingredients and directions, and you do it often. You get confident in your choices and procedures, and finally you do it without much thought. You become unconsciously competent, the whole process becomes effortless. Finally, you are cooking and eating effortlessly.

Anything that you deem worthy deserves some effort. If you decide that this has merit, decide to enjoy the journey. Set yourself enough limits so that you can learn from your mistakes. This is not the "30 Day Diet" or the "Lose Ten Pounds in 10 Days" phenomenon; this requires taking control of the rest of your inevitable maturity. Set yourself up for some leisure learning, as you stay connected to your quest to eat younger. This is not a test. There are no limits to how you can leisurely learn to take risks and play with your food until cooking becomes pure enjoyment and you are performing effortlessly

Making the Change

Once you have made the decision, expect change to be gradual, with forward and backward movement. Your mind may still be pulled towards the old methods of choosing and doing. But persistently go through our menus, refine your method of shopping, use tools that make preparation comfortable and easy, and with time you will attain competence.

Listen to your body: there are all kinds of recognizable signs. Decide what you want to focus on. Let's say you noticed you are gaining weight as the years go by. How can you make a change before it gets out of hand? There are always endless possibilities. One of the best choices would be to look at your activity and what you are eating. The menu section gives you guidelines in portion size, and the recipes provide information that could help you adjust your eating in a natural manner in order to keep a youthful, but healthy body.

Health Benefits of Eating Younger

Because body systems are interconnected, a major benefit of making a choice to eat younger is that you can automatically make a great improvement on your overall health. Over 30 years ago, Joan Borysenko wrote in her book, <u>Minding the Body, Mending the Mind,</u> about chemical messengers that are produced by the Central Nervous System, the immune system and other organs that communicate with each other to determine how we act and feel. My mood changed from hopeful to confident when I discovered this information. It was very empowering for me to realize that I had a choice, a part to play in how well I can approach aging. The ball of choice is now in your court. This is the ultimate dream of synergy. Once you decide to eat the foods that keep your immune system youthful, you are sending a message to your brain that keeps it young, delaying those senior moments of memory lapses. One of the major jobs of our immune system is to recognize and snuff out cells that are potentially cancerous. If our immune system is not getting food with essential substances that support this effort, performance of the system is lowered and diseases like cancer can occur. As we age, our systems become less efficient, so we have to be extra vigilant about our food choices. The evidence is out there that what you eat can control production of the brain chemicals that enhance mood.

Body systems also lean toward homeostasis, or balance. If you choose the right food, it keeps the acid-to-alkaline ratio in the body balanced. Loss of this balance can speed up aging. So now you have a choice to eat foods that help you put on a happier, more youthful face.

Tools for Success

One of the necessary tools for success is learning to be comfortable and confident when you are in the kitchen preparing a meal. You can build confidence by cooking on a regular basis. In this way, you would become more comfortable with various appliances and time-saving kitchen gadgets. You will also develop kitchen skills that automatically boost confidence. This will also help you to change your attitude about the time it takes to prepare a meal. Most of us have memories of our mothers or grandmothers spending hours in the kitchen just to prepare dinner, and we immediately think this is not how I want to spend my time. You might even consider how lucky you are to be able to get fast or frozen meals, but consider that you use your time waiting in lines with all the people who believe this idea saves time. But most of you give up the power of choice that determines what goes into your meal that can be of utmost benefit to you. Grandmother knew exactly what was in those meals; along with the freshest ingredients, there was a dose of love of self and family.

Cooking these recipes on a regular basis will help you to garner some of that attitude. If you use modern kitchen conveniences, like a microwave oven and food processors, you can make these meals and not be resentful of the time spent.

For chopping and cutting, you will need a chef's knife, a paring knife, boning knife and a good chopping board. If you buy good knives and a good honing instrument, you will be happier. I received kitchen scissors as a gift from one of my nieces and was amazed at how helpful they were in preparing vegetables and herbs for cooking, along with its regular uses like cutting string and cheesecloth.

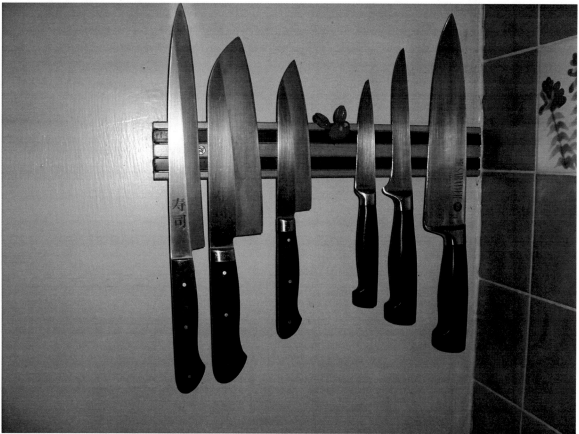

Figure 1 - Kitchen Tools

For cooking, you will need a small stockpot, one medium saucepan, one small saucepan, a steaming basket, one medium heavy-bottom skillet and one large heavy-bottom skillet.

For making dressing and salads, get large and small bowls and whisks. I also use a hand blender, which comes with its own cup or beaker and cover. This is a very convenient and quick way to make dressings and purees. These are very basic, but as you get more excited about cooking, it would be like any other hobby and you will get to know all the good kitchen stores in your area and become familiar with their stock and what suits your needs.

Collect utensils and gadgets as you perceive what you need to make this effortless. Try not to buy whole sets of anything until you find out what works for you.

Food Choices

Plan to eat seasonal fruit and vegetables. Also, try to shop around the periphery of the supermarket. Shop with a weekly menu until your new habit is sealed and you no longer crave your old way of eating. Try some of the sample menus and then make up your own. Pretty soon it becomes effortless.

This book gives you an opportunity to experiment with new foods. See what you like and what you want to add to your diet. Remember, people have been eating food like quinoa, jicama, papaya, greens like Swiss chard and kale, and fish like shark and salmon for centuries and reaping the benefits. I have avoided foods with high glycemic indexes that turn into sugar quickly and overload your system with excess sugar. The mystery of glycemic index is still being researched and there are definite believers and non-believers in this method. The book, <u>The GI Factor</u>, by Leeds, Miller, Foster-Powell and Colagiuri, gives a list of tables of popular foods and their glycemic indexes. In the meantime, I have opted for using these foods sparingly in my diet. Consequently, this book does not have many menus that that call for highly-sweetened drinks, (10-15gms or more of sugar), foods made with white flour, or sugary desserts. Also, the menus use starchy carbohydrates like baked potatoes, corn and pumpkin sparingly, so eating the right portion size should not cause weight gain or disrupt carbohydrate metabolism.

Notice your excuses and find ways to release them. Notice what you say to yourself about food. If you say, "I can't stop eating sweets" or "I am addicted to chocolate," chances are you will not talk yourself into cleaning up your act. If you make excuses after being aware that you need to make a change and don't get around to taking the right action, chances are you will continue to live by your excuses. For instance, if your excuse is "I never have time or money or help," then you will be a person who never has time to cook, shop or eat well, and you probably would not appreciate or notice when you are being helped. You may even think of advice as criticism or an insult.

Celebration, Rituals and Traditions

Life in society is made up of traditions. Usually traditions are carried out with celebration and rituals. By the time we celebrate our first birthday, we get our first taste of the foods of celebration: ice cream and cake. As we get used to the traditions of our country and ethnicity, we realize that food is a vital part of maintaining traditions. Starting with Christopher Columbus and his crew, we want to carry our food with us wherever we move, adding it to another country's own celebrations and traditions.

Celebration and traditional foods are associated with fun and comfort. I would say that most of them could even be called "fun foods" or "comfort foods." Most comfort or fun foods are made with simple carbohydrates like sugar and are combined with fats like butter, such as ice cream, cake, and pastries and chocolates. I would not even consider suggesting that you eliminate these from your diet. However, I would say consider what they represent, and notice how often in a day or a week you are seeking joy or comfort from such food. Ask yourself why and what else is possible for you to create comfort and joy on a daily basis. It's not the once-per-year Valentine or Easter candy, or the various birthdays, that can harm a balanced diet, but your daily rituals. Check and see how often in one day you reach for that sweetened drink, even if it is sugar-free. If you perceive that you are feeding your sweet tooth, you are out of the realm of celebration and into cravings or addiction with food.

Becoming aware of your problem with a certain food is the first step to easing out of such an addiction and moving towards what you want to experience for yourself. Since most of our cravings develop in childhood because of the beliefs and traditions that were imposed upon us, we unconsciously accept them as the truth. This is your chance to examine your beliefs consciously to see if it is true that the foods and traditions you are clinging to bring you comfort, joy and good health. Or, consider if you are afraid that you would be missing out on something wonderful without them. If you become aware of having a difficult time with food cravings, and can't imagine making the change you want without difficulty, you might want to seek guidance. Shakti Gawain's book, <u>Creative Visualization</u>, will help you garner the mental energy to affirm your present desires about creating the life you want now. Wayne Dyer's book, <u>Your Sacred Self</u>, will help you to see new possibilities for yourself, teach you how to notice what you do and how to change, now that you know better. With the help and guidance of these books, pretty soon the change will seem effortless.

You can even make up your own celebration menus that keep with the life you want to create in order to support your youthfulness. Since my quest for youthfulness and healthfulness, I have added a host of foods to my celebration food list, and kept some from the traditions and celebrations of my youth. I gave up toffees and jams, but I kept dark chocolate and shortbread cookies that I eat occasionally and only at teatime. *(See pg. 37 example of celebration menu)*

How We Change as We Age

We change internally at first. Little subtle changes happen in the cells of organs, like the liver, kidneys and digestive tract. Mostly we are unaware of this mishap at the cellular level until something external, like changes in skin texture or digestion happens to get our attention. We are mostly made up of billions and billions of cells equipped to do some pretty amazing things for us. For instance, we can produce progeny and keep all our internal organs and systems working together with little thought. But we must have food, energy and water. The molecules from food that our bodies can use very effectively are carbohydrates, proteins and fats. To do this, we go through a process called metabolism. This is a process of breaking down what we take in as food and using it to build what we need to be in tip-top shape. As we age, our metabolism slows down, which means we are not using all the food we eat, but instead storing it as fat and/or toxic by-products. The human thing to do is to adjust the diet with which we are familiar to one that would be more beneficial. We have come to associate this process with change, which is hard to do, and deprivation, which is discomforting, steals our joy and depresses our spirit. When we don't choose wisely we feel guilty, get stressed out about betraying ourselves, and turn to food for renewed comfort. Meanwhile, our bodies are responding to all this in many different ways, one of which is premature aging. Speaking from my experiences in my field of study, cell biology, I have witnessed under a microscope how easy it is for human cells to become stressed and age while growing in a food media that was old or not quite balanced. With this personal connection at the cellular level, I sometimes find myself thinking about what would make my cells happy, as well as what I want to eat. American Institute of Cancer Research (AICR) is constantly doing research studies on diet and disease, which reveals that eating choices are essential for excellent health, well-being and resistance to illnesses like cancer.

When we are young, our bodies are in prime shape, being supported by cells that can renew and repair tissue in organs with alarming speed. New skin cells make our faces and complexion have the glow of youth. As we age, production of enzymes, which speed things up, and the rate of food absorption start to slow down. Foods that kept us in great shape, happy and contented is now turning to fat and giving us stress. We gain weight and have new lifestyle symptoms, like high cholesterol, high blood pressure or low blood sugar. This is the beginning of aging. Your doctor tells you that you have to stop eating this kind and that kind of food. This is your first hint at the connection between food and aging. Because food is such joy, this can be very upsetting. In this book, we show the possibility of totally enjoying the rewards of food. With the use of fresh food, new preparations and portion sizes, we expand your choices with foods that will give you back your zest, appearance of youthfulness, and most of all banish that deprived feeling.

The food you eat will support your immune system, strengthen your heart and give you better brain function. I have heard people say, "I was fine until I turned 32, and then I got allergies" or "I turned 50 and then I got asthma." Changing what and how we eat as we age will keep us balanced and in good internal shape. This gives the appearance of being ageless.

A tendency today is to take an overload of vitamins or medications to target every symptom of aging that comes up. Sometimes this works, but vitamins and minerals are not a prime source of energy and can only be used properly by your body in conjunction with eating food. That is why they are called supplements. In fact, with an improper diet, an overload of supplements can act as a toxin and cause even more cellular stress. The wonder of food is that it comes with so many of its own vitamins and minerals, which work so well together it would be a shame to overlook this synergistic factor. For instance, an avocado has 17 essential minerals and vitamins, including the mineral manganese, which can substantially lower blood sugar. Here is a reason to eat your guacamole!

Change and Eating Younger Effortlessly

Before we can eat younger, we must first face the fact that mostly we eat unconsciously. We tend to eat meals and snacks that gave us comfort and joy as children. Picking up this book shows that you have good intentions. Making the recipes moves you into a conscious action. This is the dynamic start to eating with purpose, eating consciously. For this reason there are sample weekly menus as a first step, and without rigorous rules. There are no measurements of fat grams and portion sizes. The recipes serve one or two. And so you can enjoy the cooking and being with the food, no preparation time is given. Since I have made most of these recipes on a regular basis for a decade, I know they can be prepared within 30 minutes to one hour. In my experience with food, there are no bad foods, just bad choices. The choice of recipes in this book can give you the ageless edge and keep you in comfort. I once heard a lecture on nutrition from a doctor specializing in human wellness, and he said that he advises his patients to think of a serving size as a handful. He said that his patients did not understand measurement in grams. He pointed out that it is the way that they would have to do it if they were hunting and gathering. It seemed so profound at the time. I have tried it and it makes sense. You know that you are over-eating if what's on the plate seems like 3 handfuls.

In this book, there is a section on Snacks. I have found that one-half of a handful is exactly right for a snack. Try it; it is about 10-12 almonds, which I think is a great snack. You might find this very comforting. Try to consider the abundance and variety of fruit, meats, vegetables and herbs, and expand your choices. Choose food from cuisines that you have never eaten before and that have a reputation for being healthy. If you prepare them in a way that tastes good, you've just started a new tradition for your health. This book has lots of familiar foods that are prepared quickly and some with new twists to give you more pleasure in eating, and yet it keeps the balance that creates better health and less stress on your body systems.

Imbalance Nutrition and Premature Aging

Clues of premature aging show up when your body has symptoms and signs of aging that do not correspond with your actual age. I learned this lesson when I was 19 years. I went to the doctor for nausea and a host of digestive problems, and he ordered a pregnancy test because he said I was too young to have these symptoms. It turned out that after the test and some horrible stomach and colon tests, he said to me, "I wish I was reporting that you were pregnant, because the only other reason for these symptoms could be that you are stressed out and eating improperly because of your upset stomach." At the time, I was in a disgusting office atmosphere and secretly putting up with sexual harassment by the top official. Everyone was shocked when I quit my job. There goes the end of the stress. I then started my pursuit of the best nutrition for my situation, and I am still on that quest. I noticed that I feel better if I eliminate certain foods and add something that is more beneficial for me.

Imbalances in nutrition show up long before there is a crisis. It is a good thing to note why you are out of sorts, or always dealing with minor illness, or taking over-the-counter drugs for ailments that don't necessarily require a prescription. Minor symptoms like frequent indigestion, heartburn, brittle hair and nails, insomnia, proneness to yeast and fungal infections, weight gain, frequent colds, mood swings or lack of joy, lower back pain, aching joints and muscles, complexion problems, constipation, and blood sugar imbalances can be wake-up calls for you to boost your nutritional intake, before these turn into chronic aging problems.

Once you focus on eating to be younger, it will balance your internal energy and help you to resist cellular stress. Then your organ systems will perform as if they were younger and resisting aging. This change in eating can take you from feeling blue to feeling happy that you are doing something very good for your body. This shows up in your outward appearance as the traits of youthfulness, such as lots of vitality, healthy skin and nails, and an attitude that is full of joy and great expectations for life. After a while, when you become very familiar with your new eating habits, it will seem effortless to you.

Introduction to Menus

These menus get you off to a natural start. They help you explore cooking with fresh foods and making choices that support keeping yourself younger. Plan to eat seasonal fruit and red, yellow, orange and dark green vegetables. You will notice that you are mostly shopping around the periphery of the supermarket, where the fresh, uncooked and unpreserved foods are placed. Shop with a weekly menu until your new habit is sealed and you no longer crave your old way of eating. Try some of the sample menus and then make up your own from the salad, soup and dinner sections. When you have gone through a week of menus you will become familiar with how you shop and the kinds of changes you have to make to be successful at managing your new eating lifestyle. With practice, it will soon become effortless.

You will be able to compose your own menus with recipes from this book after you have established the habit of eating meals and snacks with the correct portion size that supports a healthy weight. To compose menus, use fresh food that is in season. You will notice that they will be plentiful and inexpensive. Make sure that you eat natural, non-manmade food 95% of the time.

Buy or make 100% whole grain bread, or bread with nuts and seeds, and avoid snacking on food made from white flour, like white crackers, soft pretzels, white bread, cookies and cakes. White flour is digested into sugar very quickly, starting with the enzymes in your mouth, and it can cause imbalances in insulin production. This leads to degenerative disorders like low blood sugar syndromes, and plaque formation in arteries. These disorders in metabolism can cause poor health, as well as speed up aging.

These menus help to broaden your choices, and give you the opportunity to eat regularly and stop feelings of deprivation and hunger. They are balanced so that you get enough alkaline foods like vegetables, fruits, spices, seasoning and herbal teas, along with acidic foods like meat, cereals, eggs, beans and nuts. Your body has to maintain a balanced hydrogen ion concentration (pH) between acid and alkaline. Eating twice as many alkaline foods as acidic foods will keep your diet balanced. If your blood becomes too acidic, it causes aging symptoms like changes in cartilage in joints. This can cause you to have unnecessary pain in your knees, shoulders and other joints.

As the weeks pass, notice what makes you feel less than terrific, and what has changed in your overall health. You might find that some unwanted symptoms of aging, like pain in joints or insomnia just go away. Your mood swings might disappear. It will be different for everyone, but keeping a rhythm of eating like this tends to bring your organ system into a balanced function. Just eating the right food at the right time can have an enormous effect on your brain chemistry. You don't have to do the chemistry, just eat the right combination of foods at breakfast and your brain goes to work, balancing your brain chemistry by producing neurotransmitters like serotonin, dopamine, nor epinephrine, and acetylcholine. For you this means perkiness, little or no mood swings, and a sharpened memory at work or at play!

These are not complicated menus with special types of foods, and the dietary directions are not complex. They are just what an old-fashioned, health-minded mother might recommend; three well-balanced meals a day and two snacks. If you know what you want to happen, like having better digestion, then you can pick foods that have digestive enzymes, like kiwi, papaya and pineapple. If you want to add more bulk in your diet to aid elimination, then choose foods with plenty of fiber like lentils, grains like quinoa, and whole grain bread. If you have mood swings and insomnia, get your meals and portion size back into balance, because nothing makes you age quicker than poor nutrition plus lack of sleep. This process can be quite empowering. As you pay more attention to yourself, you become more involved with knowing what is particularly right for you. This kind of experimentation with self-awareness also increases your self confidence and patience with normal life processes as you age.

About the Menus

When you are ready to get started, shop at least once per week for the firmest produce and freshest meats using a weekly menu. You will be shopping mostly for fresh food, except condiments and some canned vegetables like tomatoes, beans, coconut and soymilk, and 100% fruit or vegetable juice.

Purchase food in small quantities, since your portion sizes will be smaller and the directions on recipes serve one or two. The menus follow the recommended United States Department of Agriculture (USDA) portion size, which is actually beneficial but might seem small by American standards for serving sizes of most foods. One thing that might seem difficult is getting used to eating the portion size. If this happens, and you become hungry, wait 30 minutes and then drink herbal tea or water. Pretty soon it will be time to eat your snack for that portion of the day. This will help you to keep from over-eating and help you become aware of your feeling of fullness. In this way you will not miss eating 4 times the portion size of starchy foods like rice and pasta or meat that is usually served in restaurants.

One adjustment that will be welcome is that you get the opportunity to eat often. This will speed up your metabolic rate and help you maintain a healthy weight. For this there is a chapter on snacks. If your goal is to eat more naturally, then getting a fresh attitude will be easy since most of the recipes call for fresh food.

One of the best parts of cooking what you eat is seeking it out. This is the old ancestral urge to hunt and gather; a major game of life. You can stay in the game by making a weekly adventure of finding the freshest food at the best local markets. Attitude is everything, shop as if you are shopping for the most important person in the world and the rewards are going to be astonishing.

This ultimate energy game of seeking and gathering what is needed will revive your spirit level and allow your body and mind to reach a higher level of being.

There is a celebration menu. Most celebrations are traditionally centered on some kind of food or drink. This is a time to eat what you associate with comfort and joy, or because it has some special memory, or it is your latest and best food find. However, be cautious that you are not celebrating on your favorite food every day. This could distract you off your course for balanced eating. In any case, celebrating on a certain food every day is more of a craving than a celebration.

1st Week

Monday

Breakfast
- **One egg**
- **Sliced tomatoes with squeeze of lime, salt and pepper**
- **1 slice whole grain bread with pat of butter**

Snack
- **4 oz. fresh or 100% calcium-fortified orange juice**
- **Spring water**

Lunch
- **Soup: 1 10 oz. bowl of chili with beans**
- **Plate of Spring greens with green dressing**
- **1 slice corn bread**
- **Herb tea**

Teatime
- **Decaf green tea**
- **½ half handful of nuts**
- **3 dried apricots**

Dinner
- **4 oz. Mahi Mahi with Tomato Sauce**
- **1 cup steamed kale**
- **½ cup rice with 1 tsp. parsley pesto**

Tuesday

Breakfast
- **2 oz. Sardines**
- **1 slice whole grain toast**
- **Diced papaya with fresh cilantro, lime juice, salt and pepper sauce**

Snack
- **Fruit cup of seasonal fruit**
- **Water with lemon**

Lunch
- **1 10 oz. bowl Lentil Soup**
- **Mixed Spring greens with kiwi, green onions, walnuts and green dressing**

Teatime
- **Herb tea**
- **½ cucumber/smoked salmon sandwich**

Dinner
- **¼ Roasted chicken with gravy**
- **1 cup steamed broccoli, carrots and quinoa**

Wednesday

Breakfast
- Muscle Mania Smoothie

Snack
- ½ toast sandwich with Almond butter.
- Spring water.

Lunch
- Asian five-spice soup with chicken tenders.
- Green bean and sesame salad.

Tea-Time
- Green tea and buttered toast with fresh sliced strawberries.

Dinner
- Crab burger with power salad.

Thursday

Breakfast
- A Votre Santé Muffin with pat of butter,
- Decaf breakfast tea.

Snack
- 6 oz. calcium-fortified soymilk or 4 oz. 100% juice.

Lunch
- Tabouli salad with ½ cup sliced roasted chicken.
- Spring water.

Tea-Time
- Herb tea, cup of melon.

Dinner
- Curried shrimp with ½ cup basmati rice,
- Mixed salad greens with diced apple, walnuts and red onion and honey mustard dressing.

Friday

Breakfast
- Larry's Corn Bread with butter
- Tablespoon sun dried tomatoes in oil.
- ½ grapefruit.

Snack
- Your favorite apple
- 1 bottle spring water

Lunch
- Cucumber Raita
- 2 handfuls of Stone ground tortilla chips
- Tomato salsa

Tea Time
- Decaffeinated Green Tea
- Handful cranberries and 2 squares of 70% dark chocolate

Dinner
- Linguine with baby Clams
- Sautéed shitake mushrooms with steamed kale
- Carrot Salad

Saturday

Breakfast
- A votre santé muffin with almond butter
- Small navel orange
- Coffee

Snack
- 1 Handful roasted mixed dry nuts
- Spring water

Lunch
- Chili with beans
- Sliced avocado with Squeeze of fresh lime juice

Tea-time
- Short bread cookie with dried apricots
- Herb tea

Dinner
- Grilled salmon with apple dill rosemary sauce
- Cinco de Mayo salad
- Steamed rice
- Grilled mixed vegetables

Sunday

Breakfast
- Sardines with diced tomatoes and green onions
- High fiber (3 gm or more)whole grain toast
- Coffee or tea

Snack
- 6 oz. calcium fortified and vitamin D orange juice
- 1 handful nuts and seeds

Lunch
- Shrimp and artichoke salad
- Toasted whole grain bread with extra virgin olive oil
- Mineral water

Tea-time
- Decaffeinated tea
- Whole grain crackers with parsley pesto and goat cheese

Dinner
- 1 cup of cream of butternut squash soup
- Roasted Cornish hens with sweet red pepper sauce
- Basmati rice
- steamed green beans and sliced red onions with a dash of extra virgin olive oil and balsamic vinegar
- Yoghurt with fresh mixed berries

2nd
Week

Monday

Breakfast
- Quick eggs, sliced tomatoes, squeeze of lime, salt and pepper.
- 1 slice whole grain bread with pat of butter.

Snack
- 4 oz. calcium-fortified juice.
- Spring water.

Lunch
- Soup –1 10 oz. bowl of chili with beans.
- Carrot Salad.

Tea-Time
- Decaf green tea, ½ handful of nuts.

Dinner
- 4 oz. Mahi-Mahi Fish with tomato sauce,
- Steamed kale,
- ½ cup rice with 1tsp. parsley pesto.

Tuesday

Breakfast
- Sardines and whole grain toast,
- Diced papaya with cilantro and pepper sauce.

Snack
- 1 orange.
- Water with lemon.

Lunch
- 1 10 oz. bowl Lentil Soup,
- Mixed spring greens with kiwi, green onions and walnuts.

Tea-Time
- Herb tea,
- ½ cucumber/smoked salmon sandwich.

Dinner
- ¼ Roasted chicken with au jus sauce,
- Steamed broccoli, carrots and quinoa.

Wednesday

Breakfast
- Muscle Mania Smoothie.

Snack
- ½ toast sandwich with Almond butter.
- Spring water.

Lunch
- Asian five-spice soup.
- Green bean and sesame salad.

Tea-Time
- Green tea and buttered toast with strawberries.

Dinner
- Crab burger with power salad.

Thursday

Breakfast
- A Votre Sante Muffin with pat of butter,
- Decaf breakfast tea,
- 6 oz. plain yogurt with fresh fruit.

Snack
- 6 oz. calcium-fortified soymilk or 4 oz. juice.

Lunch
- Tabouli salad with ½ cup sliced roasted chicken.

Tea-Time
- Herb tea,
- Cup of melon.

Dinner
- Curried shrimp with ½ cup basmati rice,
- Mixed salad greens with avocado,
- Kiwi and honey mustard dressing.

Friday

Breakfast
- Berry Good smoothie.

Snack
- 1 slice whole grain toast with fresh goat cheese.
- Spring water.

Lunch
- 10 oz. bowl of Lucian broth,
- Carrot salad.

Tea-Time
- Decaf green tea,
- ½ half handful of almonds.

Dinner
- Grilled pork chops with red pepper sauce,
- Steamed broccoli and,
- 1 cup thin spaghetti.

Saturday

Breakfast
- Mushroom omelet,
- Whole grain toast,
- Diced papaya with cilantro and hot sauce.

Snack
- 1 cup fruit in season.
- Spring water with lemon.

Lunch
- 1 cup cilantro potato salad with sliced roast chicken and salad greens.

Tea-Time
- Herb tea,
- Hummus with toasted Pita.

Dinner
- Grilled salmon with orange sauce,
- Baby sweet peas,
- Diced carrots and quinoa.

Sunday

Breakfast
- Baked apple with breakfast pork chops.

Snack
- One cup of seasonal fruit,
- Spring water.

Lunch
- Black-eyed pea salad and corn bread,
- Herbal iced-tea.

Tea-Time
- Green tea and buttered toast with fresh strawberries.

Dinner
- Callaloo soup with ½ cup rice,
- Sea scallops with tomato sauce,
- Papaya mandarin salad

3rd

Week

Monday

Breakfast
- Fortified cereal, with ¼ cup dried apricots,
- 6 oz. low-carbohydrate soymilk.

Snack
- 1 oz. cheese on 1 slice 100% whole grain bread.
- Spring water.

Lunch
- Soup –1 10 oz. bowl Asian soup with chicken.
- Papaya salad.

Tea-Time
- Decaf green tea,
- ½ half handful of pumpkin seeds,
- Small green apple.

Dinner
- Strawberry spinach salad,
- Baked Red Snapper with tomato sauce,
- Steamed asparagus and ½ cup quinoa.

Tuesday

Breakfast
- Veggie Breakfast quesadilla with tomato salsa,
- Decaf coffee.

Snack
- 6 oz. calcium-fortified orange juice.

Lunch
- 1 medium plate of shrimp,
- Artichoke salad,
- 1 cup cream of butternut squash soup.

Tea-Time
- Herb tea,
- Pita chips with hummus and parsley pesto.

Dinner
- Gazpacho,
- Potato frittata,
- Warm broccoli and asparagus salad.

Wednesday

Breakfast
- Quick eggs,
- Papaya salsa with corn tortillas.

Snack
- Mixed fresh fruit with chopped almonds.
- Spring water.

Lunch
- 10 oz. bowl of chili bean soup with diced onions
- Corn bread.

Tea-Time
- Green tea,
- Cucumber sandwich with smoked salmon.

Dinner
- ½ Cornish Hen,
- Tabouli salad and,
- Steamed bok choy and carrots.

Thursday

Breakfast
- Strawberry Smoothie.

Snack
- ½ sandwich with almond butter.
- Spring water.

Lunch
- Curried chicken salad,
- 1 cup of onion soup.

Tea-Time
- Herb tea,
- 1 apple,
- ½ handful pumpkin seeds.

Dinner
- Linguine with clam sauce,
- Power salad.

Friday

Breakfast
- **Breakfast pork chop,**
- **1 slice whole grain toast with butter,**
- **Pineapple and strawberry fruit cup.**

Snack
- **1 handful pumpkin seeds.**
- **Spring water.**

Lunch
- **10 oz. bowl of Avocado soup,**
- **Stone-ground corn chips and tomato salsa.**

Tea-Time
- **Decaf green tea,**
- **¼ cup dried mixed fruit.**

Dinner
- **Grilled White fish with tomato sauce,**
- **Steamed rice with grated carrots,**
- **Warm broccoli and asparagus salad.**

Saturday

Breakfast
- **Smoothie with low-carbohydrate protein powder.**

Snack
- **1 open-faced smoke salmon and cucumber sandwich,**
- **Spring water with fresh lime.**

Lunch
- **1 cup chicken salad on mixed greens, baked apple.**

Tea-Time
- **Herb tea,**
- **Mini scones with goat cheese.**

Dinner
- **Caramelized Quail,**
- **Grilled mixed vegetables,**
- **Asian soup with shiitake mushrooms and,**
- **Steamed rice.**

Sunday

Breakfast
- Salted cod with tomatoes and eggs,
- Toasted pita,
- Coffee or tea.

Snack
- 6 oz. calcium-fortified orange juice,
- ½ handful nuts and seeds.

Make up your own menu. Use your special food combination from this book.

Keep it balanced with protein, fat and fiber thinking about the mineral, vitamins and antioxidants for your special needs.

Lunch
- Lentil soup with feta cheese,
- Toasted whole grain bread with herb olive oil and,
- Green tea.

Tea-Time
- Decaf tea and buttered toast,
- Fresh strawberries.

Dinner
- 1 cup chicken tortilla soup,
- Shrimp curry with vegetables,
- Basmati rice,
- Yogurt with fresh mixed berries.

Celebration Menu

- **Cream of butternut squash soup with your favorite crackers.**
- **Caramelized Quail on a bed of strawberry-spinach salad with fresh honey mustard dressing.**
- **Shepherds pie with steamed asparagus and onions.**
- **Sourdough bread or pita chips with parsley pesto, herb olive oil or butter.**
- **Baked apple with frozen chocolate yogurt and chopped walnuts.**
- **Your favorite white wine.**

EatYounger Breakfast

Breakfast Series

This is your chance to seize the day, to energize and keep your nutritional intentions active. Breakfast can give you the edge at work, give housewives stamina and add many more beautiful healthy years to your life. This is your first chance to attack premature or accelerated aging and start a more successful ritual at the beginning of your day.

Skipping breakfast is like trying to get your car to start without fuel. Unfortunately, our bodies are not tied to mechanical devices. We have a mind that can override our decision to skip breakfast and keep us moving on to what we perceive as the next logical step. In your case, you might be moving, but vital processes and pathways are at a standstill internally.

When you choose wisely for breakfast, you can jumpstart body systems like your central nervous and vascular systems and keep them younger. While others are sniffling, your immune system will be on the alert, catching mishaps and resisting disease with ease. You will resist blood sugar imbalances like hypo or hyperglycemia. Your heart will be happier and healthier because you did the right thing and your blood vessels will stay unclogged.

The effect of skipping breakfast and trying to operate without fuel, which for us is carbohydrates, proteins and fats, will not show up for years. We notice it when we have symptoms of aging.

You can use breakfast as your chance to rev up your metabolic rate, stay as young as you desire, and stop leaning on a cup of coffee, a powerful stimulant, to do the job. Although coffee does a good job of waking you up and getting you ready for the fray of the day, it could be a false start if you did not have other vital nutrients like amino-acids from protein, and fatty acids from fats, to keep your brain cells nourished while the caffeine stimulation is happening. Without this, you soon become addicted to coffee, your cravings increase with frequent use and you experience withdrawal symptoms when you try to do without it.

A More Successful Ritual for the Start of Your Day

Creating a ritual for breakfast
If you cling to the old way of starting your day, you will not experience success. Even worse than not eating breakfast is making choices that have little benefit or may be detrimental.

In this transition phase, *first notice what you do in the morning.* This gives you clues to what rituals you have established and what you resist when you choose to eat differently. Do not judge yourself as to your progress at this time. *To keep your intentions to make a change, you will have to replace these rituals with new ones.*

For instance, all rituals have timing and require preparation. So you might find yourself with no time as an excuse. Out of this you will create a new ritual. Noticing your thoughts is a very powerful technique that can speed up desired change. Notice the excuses you are making and resolve to stop having that excuse. As an example, if your excuse is that you never have time. Resolve to do something that will give you more time, like setting your alarm at an earlier time. Or better yet, have what you need out and ready the night before so that you use minimum time in completing the meal. Rituals also require new thought patterns, so tell yourself what great nourishment and healing you will get from this change. You can also visualize on a regular basis how well you will look and all the great compliments you will receive from being so efficient at work, or how much more energy you will have in the morning. This helps you to move with little effort into the new idea to have more time to get breakfast.

You can also create some pre-ritual activity. Clean out your fridge and pantry. This is the beginning of cleaning out your digestive system, your blood stream and exciting your mind to accept a new ritual. As you go along, read labels. Look for foods that are high in sugars such as lactose, glucose, fructose, galactose, cornstarch and high fructose corn syrup. These would be the first or second words on the ingredients list. Discard or give them away. Most jams, jellies, and juice drinks will be in your giveaway pile. Drink only 100% juice, with labels that say no sugar added. Use a small glass that would hold about six ounces. The ideal would be to only drink fresh squeezed juice.

Discard all breakfast cereals that have more than 9 grams of sugar on the label and opt for fortified, low-sugar, high-fiber breakfast cereals. This is very scary to do, so be prepared to go through many emotions and doubts. Whenever you get too scared to follow through with your intentions, think about how wonderful it would be for you not to have body aches, mood swings, food addictions, wrinkles or whatever else is your goal. These processes will increase your feeling of readiness for the new anti-aging breakfast ritual.

The breakfasts in this book are quick, and there is a healthy variety. The portion size is just enough to get you to your next meal or snack without gaining an ounce. They are the kinds of foods that sustain good health and vitality and help your body to resist aging.

To ease into the new ritual, use one of the weekly menus and purchase enough food to last for one week. Plan on shopping once per week until you are sure that you have adopted the new breakfast ritual and you don't have to think about it to be on target.

A Votre Santé Muffin

We are all aware that muffins can be the ultimate "lead you astray" food. It is quite easy to get half your daily saturated fat and sugar from one breakfast muffin, and lose your goal for balance. And who wants a muffin that is healthy but tasteless? To keep the balancing act going, these tasty muffins are low in refined sugar, but get some sweetness from the raisins or dried fruit of your choice. Dried apricots, cranberries, fresh ripe bananas, apples or strawberries can be used to replace white raisins. The wheat germ provides fiber, as well as age-retarding vitamin E and folic acid for quick cell renewal. Make this muffin a habit and you might never need to take a calcium channel blocker. The magnesium from almonds and soy milk provide natural calcium channel blocker activity for veins and arteries. Added to this, almonds contain electrolyte potassium to aid your heart and perfect nerve transmission. Canola oil is used to help you start the day with your fair share of low-density lipoproteins (LDL). The LDL health benefits of this oil can now be claimed on food labels as aiding in reducing the risk of coronary heart disease.

Ingredients

1 ½ cups whole wheat flour
½ cup wheat germ or ½ cup freshly ground flax seeds
2 tsp. baking powder
½ tsp. salt
1/3 cup brown sugar
2/3 cup sultana or white raisins
½ cup sliced almonds
1 tsp. apple pie spice and ½ tsp. freshly grated nutmeg
1 large egg and 1 large egg white
½ cup canola oil
1 cup low-sugar, calcium-fortified soy milk
1 tsp. almond extract

Steps

↳Preheat the oven to 400 F.

↳Grease muffin pans with spray vegetable oil.

↳Into a large bowl sift together the flour, wheat germ or ground flax seed, baking powder, spice and salt.

↳Spray the raisins with water and plump in a microwave oven for 15 seconds and add to the flour mixture.

↳Add the nuts to the bowl.

↳In a blender mix the egg, oil, milk and almond extract for 10 seconds.

↳Make a well in the dry ingredients in the bowl and add the wet ingredients. Gently fold wet ingredient into the dry until just mixed.

↳Spoon the mixture into greased muffin tins and bake 25-30 minutes.

↳Serve warm or cool. Can freeze for up to 1 month.

Makes 8 regular-size muffins. Serving size is one muffin.

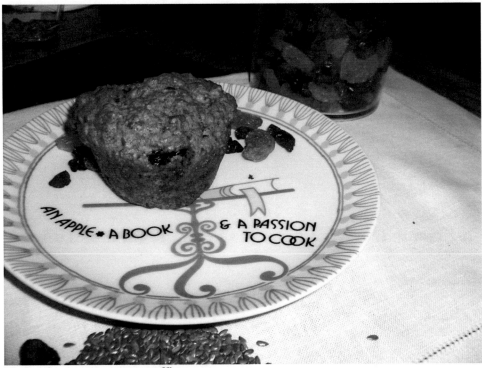

Figure 2 - A votre sante muffin

Almond Smoothie

The almond butter in this smoothie keeps the heart healthy and circulation good. Here is a lightening quick way for you to load up on some good essential oils, potent antioxidants and vitamin E. Note some of the gifts of almond butter. Almond butter has both flavonoids in its skin as well as vitamin E in its meat. This creates a huge synergistic protective benefit to slow the aging of your circulatory system. Added to this, research studies have also proven that almond butter can reduce the glycemic index (GI) of a high carbohydrate meal by lowering blood sugar levels. So if you are battling diabetes, cease the fight and relax with this smoothie. This can bring a whole new level of health, just because of your quest to eat yourself younger. Admit it, this smoothie is effortless. With the power of a high-speed blender, you are looking at 10-15 seconds after gathering ingredients.

Ingredients

4 oz. low-carbohydrate (less than 8 gm.), calcium-fortified plain soy milk
1 tbs. smooth almond butter
½ banana, sliced and frozen
3 ice cubes or 3 ounces of cold water
Dash almond extract

Steps

⟵⟶

↪Pour milk into a blender. Add almond butter, banana and other ingredients.
↪Blend until smooth.
↪Enjoy.

Baked Apples

Enjoy on whole grain toast or with plain yogurt sprinkled with wheat germ. For a more elaborate meal, eat with the breakfast pork chops recipe in this book.
This breakfast is fast. This also makes a great snack or dessert when served with a scoop of frozen yogurt. Pears can also be fixed this way.

Ingredients

1 Fuji apple, peeled and cored
1 tsp. brown sugar
Sprinkle of cinnamon
Sprinkle of nutmeg, or ¼ tsp. apple pie spice instead of cinnamon and nutmeg

Steps

↪Slice apple in ¼-inch slices.

↪Sprinkle with brown sugar and spices.

↪Bake in microwave at half-power for 1 minute, and then full-power for 30 seconds. Baking times may vary according to the strength of your oven.

Berry Good Smoothie

Make this is a salute to you and all the good things you do for your body. Buy organic blueberries and raspberries when they are in their peak season from June through September. Sort your berries and remove any that are soft, moldy or just spoiled. Wash, dry and freeze in a plastic container. Berries bring neutralization to free radicals, help stabilize collagen in cells and tissues and support the vascular system. Isn't this another answer for facial firmness? Studies about the health benefits of berries have revealed that their natural antioxidants can protect the brain from aging diseases like Alzheimer's and might even enhance memory. So with this 'berry good' habit, you might never experience a senior moment!

Ingredients

½ cup fresh frozen blueberries
½ cup fresh frozen raspberries
1 tbs. honey
6 oz. soy milk or low-fat plain yogurt
1 tsp. vanilla extract
3 ice cubes

Steps

⇦————————————————————————————⇨

↳Place milk and honey in a blender. Add berries and ice. Blend until smooth.
↳Strain if you don't want the seeds.
↳Enjoy.

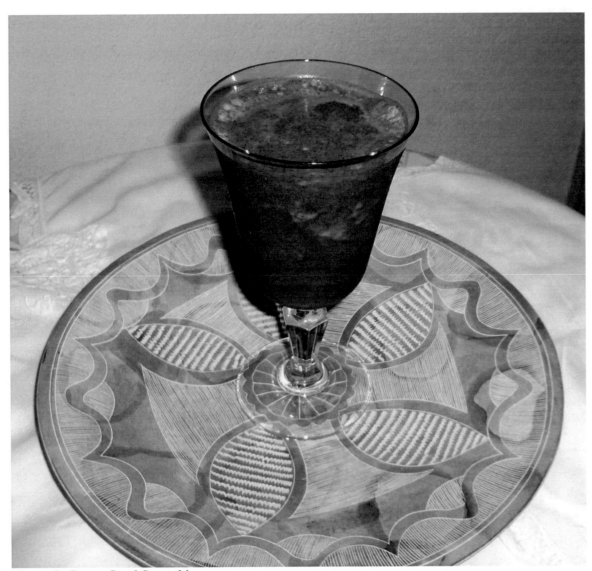

Figure 3 - Berry Good Smoothie

Breakfast Cheesy Tortilla with Salsa

This Mexican-style breakfast is served with salsa. Make the salsa beforehand so that you can have it ready for the morning. This is a very versatile salsa recipe. It can be used for other snacks, soups and dressings, and will keep in the refrigerator for 7 days. The oil of the avocado is very good for aging skin and the fruit is loaded with essential minerals and vitamins, and a substance that stabilizes blood sugar.

Ingredients

½ Hass avocado
2 small corn tortillas
4 tbs. grated Monterey Jack cheese
2 tbs. chopped green onions
Salt and pepper
Salsa: 1 14.5oz. can Mexican-style stewed tomatoes
1 fresh jalapeno pepper
Juice of ½ lime
3 tbs. fresh cilantro leaves
½ tsp salt

Steps

↬Place the tortillas on a heated large, heavy-bottom skillet or iron skillet; sprinkle 2 tbs. cheese and half of the green onions on each. Use tongs to keep turning the tortilla as it is heating. Grill until the cheese is melted. Takes about 1-2 minutes.

↬To make the salsa, put ¼ of the tomatoes, cilantro, the pepper, salt and limejuice in a food processor. Pulse and mix gently until all ingredients are mixed. Then add the rest of the tomatoes and mix for about 10 seconds until all ingredients are chopped. Pour into a glass container and store.

↬Slice the avocado while it is still in the skin. Scoop out the slices onto a serving dish and serve with salsa and the cheesy tortillas.

↬Enjoy.

Tropical Dreams Smoothie

This is a real pick-me-up. Make this smoothie when you really want to be somewhere warm and wonderful in the winter. Guava nectars are available in leading grocery stores in small bottles or 12 oz. cans. Buy pineapples when they are in season, peel and cut into small pieces and freeze in plastic freezer bags or containers. Guavas have a bioactive substance that is beneficial to healthy prostate function. Pineapples are high in manganese, a trace mineral which supports the energy-producing packets of human cells called mitochondria. This smoothie slows aging as it brings more vim and vigor for you.

Ingredients

½ cup guava nectar
1 tsp. fresh lime juice
½ cup fresh frozen pineapple
½ cup plain low-fat yogurt
5 ice cubes

Steps

⮜⮞

🖎Add the nectar and lime juice to a blender.
🖎Add the pineapple and all other ingredients.
🖎Blend until smooth.
🖎A half-serving of lactose-free, low-sugar protein powder would make this a balanced breakfast meal. Use a low-carbohydrate (1 gram) whey protein that mixes instantly with liquids. Add the protein powder after the smoothie is blended but still in the blender. When added, stir it in on the lowest setting of the blender.

Larry's Corn Bread

If you want to avoid yeast bread and still pack in some serious nourishment, choose corn. This bread is packed full of B vitamins and folate. It can be a complete breakfast with mixed fruit, or sliced tomatoes and green onions. The beautiful thing about this bread is that it has grains and protein in one remarkable slice. Not only is the yogurt providing protein, but also it will boost your calcium intake. Corn supports lung health through a carotenoid called beta-cryptoxanthin and memory with thiamin, vitamin B1.

Ingredients

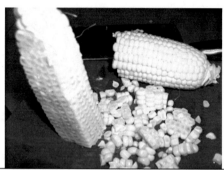

1 cup of frozen corn, or kernels from 2 ears of freshly-cooked corn
¼ cup of canola oil
1 large egg and 2 egg whites
1 cup plain non-fat yogurt
1 cup soymilk
2 tbs. whipping cream (optional)
4 green onions
1 Jalapeno pepper, seeds removed (optional)
2 cups stone ground cornmeal
2 tsp. baking powder
½ tsp. salt
½ cup grated Monterey Jack cheese
½ cup of white cheddar

Steps

↰—————————————————————————————————→

↳Preheat oven to 325 F. Spray a large pie plate or 9-inch square baking dish with olive oil cooking spray.

↳Cook the frozen corn in the microwave for 2 minutes or cook the fresh corn in a microwave dish with 1 tbs. of water for 2 minutes. Let cool, and then remove the kernels by cutting lengthways with a sharp knife.

↳Using a blender mix the oil, eggs, yogurt, milk, corn, cream, green onions and pepper until liquefied, about 10 seconds.

↳Place the cornmeal, baking powder and salt in a large mixing bowl.

↳Mix dry ingredients with wet until incorporated.

↳Pour half of mixture into the greased container. Combine the grated cheeses, and then add half of the cheese mixture.

↳Pour remaining mixture over cheese. Add the rest of the cheese.

↳Bake 45 minutes until a toothpick inserted into the center comes out clean.

↳Remove from oven and let cool. This bread will last in the fridge for 1 week or can be frozen for up to 1 month.

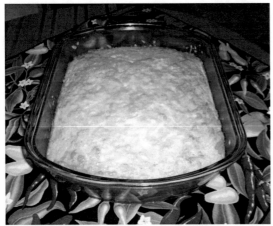
Figure 4 - Freshly baked corn bread

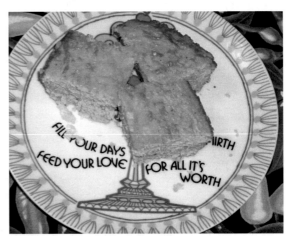
Figure 5 - Sliced Corn Bread

Mango Smoothie

Mangoes are the quintessential tropical fruit. They are found in abundance in tropical landscapes. The fruit is used green or ripe. The ripe fruit is quite sweet. There are many varieties and they all have distinctive flavors. Store-bought mangoes can be kept at room temperature until ready for use. They can also be cut up and frozen for use in smoothies. This smoothie is the next best thing to a fresh pick. To make this smoothie, freeze the ripe fruit after it is peeled and the large seed has been removed. Mangoes are rich in vitamins A and C. This smoothie has a comforting sunshine yellow color. Color is also an indication of its beta-carotene content, which delivers natural antioxidant action and gives you a reduction in free radicals. Because mangoes bring an alkaline quality to body fluids, it helps to keep blood fluids out of the acid range. This is excellent for anti-aging because neutrality reigns. This quick drink is a daily fresh start to lowering aging activity internally. Expect to look and feel great for a long time.

Ingredients

½ cup fresh frozen mango pieces
4 oz. vitamin D-fortified orange juice
¼ cup plain non-fat yogurt
½ tsp. vanilla extract
3 to 5 ice cubes
1 tbs. of honey, if you want a sweeter drink

Steps

⬅————————————————————————➡

↳Put ingredients in a blender, starting with the liquids first. Blend until smooth about 20 seconds.
↳Enjoy, especially when mangoes are in season.

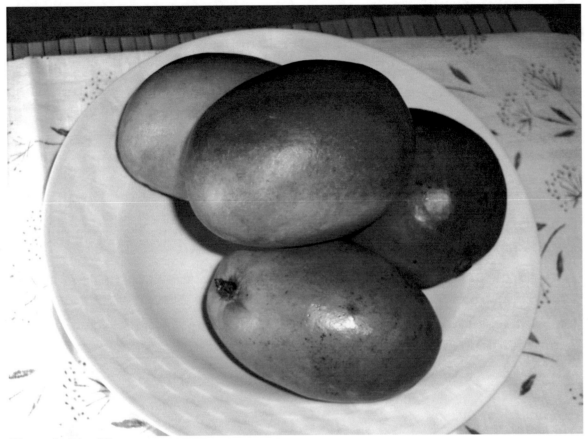

Figure 6 - Ripe Mangoes

Muscle Mania Smoothie

Gulp this smoothie down when you are going to the gym and you expect real results. It has enough carbohydrates to keep your energy up during workouts. It is high in protein, with ample potassium and chocolate to get your endorphins moving. This means that your mood will be in high gear naturally. Your muscles will be ready to work and reward you for it. As a breakfast meal, this can lift your mood for most of the day.

Ingredients

1 cup low-carbohydrate, (less than 5 gm) calcium-fortified soy milk
¼ cup frozen chocolate or coffee yogurt
1 banana, frozen and sliced
1 scoop low-carbohydrate (less than 1 gm) protein powder
Dash vanilla or almond extract

Steps

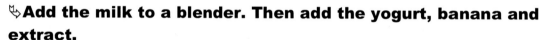

✍Add the milk to a blender. Then add the yogurt, banana and extract.
✍Blend until smooth.
✍With the blender on low, mix in the protein powder until combined.

Mushroom Omelet

If you are stressed out, this breakfast can rescue you. It will keep you recharged and your immune system ready for defense. This translates into no minor infections, and you will lose the rundown look. Your true beauty will resurface. Clean the mushrooms by wiping with a damp cloth.

Ingredients

2 large egg whites and 1 yolk
4 cleaned, sliced shiitake mushrooms
2 finely chopped green onions
2 tsp. canola oil or ghee (see ghee recipe in this book)
Sprinkling of salt, pepper and garlic powder

Steps

⟵————————————————————————————————⟶

✎Heat the oil in a small skillet. Add the onions and mushrooms and stir-fry for one minute, then cover and let the mushrooms cook for 2 – 3 minutes.

✎Whisk the eggs with salt, pepper and garlic.

✎Uncover the skillet and add the eggs. Cook over medium heat. Using a spatula move the top layer of eggs to the bottom until the eggs are evenly cooked.

✎Flip the omelet over and remove from the heat.

✎Eat with sliced tomatoes and fresh basil, or fruit of your choice.

Pork Chops and Melon

Breakfast can help you move mountains and feel ready for whatever comes along. Pork is high in lysine, an essential amino acid that helps to heal skin ailments and keep it beautiful. Lysine also supports your immune system and helps you resist and overcome viral infections. Breakfast pork chops are thin and cook more quickly than bacon. American pork is now as lean as chicken breasts, and chops will have less saturated fat than bacon. The feeling that you did something good for yourself will linger all day.

Melon is high in antioxidants to fight those free radicals, which can do untold damage to your cells. If you have been skipping breakfast, this is how you can start a new, healthy habit. You will be amazed at how well you will feel. If you tend to have a low red blood cell count, then this breakfast will give you positive results.

Ingredients

¼ lb. breakfast pork chops, thinly sliced
½ tsp. granulated garlic and ½ tsp. onion powder
1 tsp. extra virgin olive oil
Salt and pepper to taste
1 cup fresh melon, cut into small cubes

Steps

↪Brush the chops on both sides with olive oil and sprinkle with the seasonings.

↪Bake in the microwave on medium power for 1 to 2 minutes, or cook in a non-stick skillet sprayed with cooking oil over medium heat. Brown on both sides until chops are cooked but tender, about 1 ½ to 2 minutes on both sides.

↪Place on a plate, add a condiment like Pickapeppa, chili sauce or your favorite chutney, and enjoy with the fruit.

Quick Eggs

Eat this breakfast 3 times a week if you are serious about losing weight. It is fast and easy to prepare. It gives you protein and fat to keep you brain nourished, plus your body will better learn to burn fat. Since the tomato is a non-starchy carbohydrate, your blood sugar should stay stable and you will feel satisfied until your next snack. This breakfast is a good balance of acidic and alkaline foods. It is reported that balancing acidic foods with alkaline foods will help the biochemistry of your whole body to achieve a healthy balance.

Ingredients

1 jumbo egg
1 small tomato, sliced
¼ tsp. of olive oil or grape-seed oil
Sprinkle of your favorite dried herb
Salt and pepper to taste
Hot herbal tea

Steps

⟵――――――――――――――――――――――――――――――⟶

↳**Crack egg in a ramekin dish sprayed with vegetable cooking spray, grape-seed or olive oil.**
↳**Puncture yoke of egg with a toothpick in 4 different places or use a fork.**
↳**Cover and microwave for 45 seconds to 1 minute on half power.**
↳**Turn out on a plate and serve with sliced tomatoes.**
↳**Sprinkle tomatoes with salt and pepper and dried herb.**
↳**Serve with hot herbal tea and ENJOY!**

Salted Cod or Buljol

Say "hurrah" to real survival food. The slaves in the Caribbean ate this to carry them through the day. This is so satisfying that it is still a favorite breakfast of Caribbean people. The wisdom of this meal is that it brings balance to the start of your day. The fish will give you enough B vitamins to carry you through your morning and the vegetables are a good way to get minerals and vitamins. Salted cod is sold in 1 lb. boxes in most supermarkets. The fish will have to be re-hydrated with hot water, after which it will regain its flakiness and taste like fish seasoned with salt.

Ingredients

¼ lb. salted cod
1 Roma tomato, seeded and diced
½ small onion, sliced
¼ cup diced green pepper
1 hard-boiled egg, finely chopped or grated
Dash of hot pepper sauce
2 tbs. extra virgin olive oil
Juice of one small lime

Steps

⇔Break the fish into small pieces and place in a bowl. Add hot water and soak to remove the salt. Pour off the water as the salt leeches out. Repeat until the water is no longer very salty. This can be done the night before.

⇔Place the fish in a serving dish, and then add the remaining ingredients. Mix well.

⇔Serve with chopped, hard-boiled egg and sourdough French rolls.

⇔Serves one or two. Seize the day!

Sardines and Toast

Go ahead, start a tradition with this breakfast! It gives you what you are looking for: more calcium. I call this my "big Ca+ breakfast." Sardines are naturally high in omega-3 fatty acids, which have been proven to keep your heart youthful. This is a protein-rich meal. The corresponding amino acids will wake up your whole self. The tomatoes and green onion give you a fresh start with vitamin C. The whole grain toast balances out the meal with fiber. Plus, it is fast and easy.

Ingredients

1 3 oz. can sardines
2 green onions, finely chopped
1 small tomato, sliced thinly
1 tsp. lime juice or balsamic vinegar
Sprinkle of lemon pepper
1 slice whole grain toast (label should show 3 or more grams of fiber)

Steps

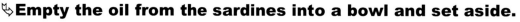

↳Empty the oil from the sardines into a bowl and set aside.
↳Place the sliced tomatoes on the bottom of a serving dish. Spread the sardines on top and garnish with the chopped onions.
↳Mix the lime juice or vinegar and the lemon pepper with the reserved oil or fresh extra virgin olive oil.
↳Pour oil over the prepared dish.
↳Eat with toast.
↳Serves two.

Hi – C Start Your Engines Smoothie

This is as good as it gets for a high-powered, quick-to-prepare breakfast. A good blender and a tall glass and you are ready. This recipe uses fresh, frozen fruit in season, fresh juice, high quality non-fat yogurt and a blender. This breakfast gives you a head start on phytochemicals like vitamin C and a substance called ellagic acid in the strawberries, which has been proven to prevent tumor formation. You will have at least three of your daily servings of fruit all in one easy meal. So why fight aging diseases like cancer when it is so much fun to prevent it? This smoothie will also increase your potassium, and add to your intake of folate by 15%. The fiber and the protein from the yogurt help to balance sugar absorption. This is a fast way to get your body systems revved up in the morning.

Ingredients

½ banana, frozen and sliced
6 medium frozen strawberries, hulled and sliced
4 oz. calcium-fortified orange juice
4 oz. plain low-fat yogurt
Dash of vanilla and honey to taste

Steps

⇆Pour the orange juice into a blender.

⇆Measure and add the yogurt.

⇆Add the frozen fruit and blend according to the directions of the manufacturer of your blender.

⇆Blend until smooth. A high-powered blender can do this in 10-12 seconds.

EatYounger Snacks

Snacks

The right snacks can keep your metabolic fires going. This means that you can expect your body to use up your meals instead of turning them into fat. Most of all, snacks help keep you from feeling deprived and hungry.

The main danger with snacks is choosing those that are commercially available, such as candy, cookies, pretzels and soft drinks, from vendor machines or quick stop stores. These kinds of snacks also tend to be unbalanced, having more sugar, salt or fat than is beneficial for slow aging. With a little planning, you can have nourishing snacks that give you just what your body needs to keep your metabolic rate and mental energy up and protect you from rapid aging. Yes, it is possible to eat snacks and not gain weight or disrupt the function of body systems. Another danger is having such a large portion of a snack that it turns into a meal. This can also cause weight gain, especially in your middle or tummy, if you choose snacks and drinks that are high in simple sugars.

Choose snacks that are not man-made for convenience or prepackaged with ingredients that improve shelf life, but instead are fresh and ready to eat. Fresh fruits, dried fruit and nuts make great snacks and have vitamins like A and C and minerals that boost your immune system.

The recipes in this section help you to prepare and choose snacks that are healthy and will maintain youthfulness. Without a plan and a ready snack, snacking can get to be detrimental. Making poor choices in snacks can lead to imbalances in fats and sugars, which can disrupt your health in general.

If you are concerned about obesity, it is possible that you might have to make only one life change, and that is in the way you choose to snack. Grabbing a soda and a host of convenience type food that is not freshly prepared is not the way to go. If you have limited time to cook, you can prepare a simple snack of fresh and dried fruit and nuts. These "grab and go" snacks are ideal, if they are eaten in the correct portion size. For instance, a dozen almonds have an omega-3 fat, which is excellent for your skin, a small amount of protein, some fiber, minerals like calcium and magnesium, vitamin E and no sugar. However, more than a dozen is snack overload. A simple apple will give you enough pectin to help you feel full and at the same time add some soluble fiber to your diet.

Making faulty choices with snacks can cause premature aging. Choosing convenience type snacks that are overloaded with sugar or saturated fat leads to poor health sugar syndromes, where there is either too much or too little insulin in your blood. When your cells are exposed to an overload of insulin they become damaged and this leads to premature aging. This is your chance to bypass all that and get in the habit of choosing a delicious, well-balanced snack in the first place. This takes some planning.

The recipes here have balanced protein, fats, and carbohydrates and are high in fiber, essential vitamins and minerals to help make your skin glow, keep you slim, boost your vitality and give you that energetic feeling of youthfulness. So turn on the enthusiasm and dump the excuses. A little bit of planning on a daily basis and it effortlessly becomes part of your daily routine. A good snack should maintain your energy level, but not overload your metabolic or food burning pathways and cause your body to turn extra food into fat so you gain weight, or worse yet, dump toxic by-products in your blood stream.

The snacks in this book are chosen because they give you extra benefits when you choose to snack. They taste good, and some of them are just plain satisfying and comforting.
Most of them are simple to prepare using a food processor and some good kitchen tools. There are snacks for when you want to celebrate, gather with friends and indulge yourself, or when you just want to have a traditional afternoon tea. Snack time should be a happy time for you, not one laden with guilt because you always make poor choices, so start snacking and get rid of the guilt.

Afternoon Tea

One of the most pleasurable things that you can do for yourself is to start a new habit of having afternoon tea as one of your snacks. The idea is to make teatime, which is generally in the late afternoon, part of your day wherever you are. This is actually a very ancient custom. The Japanese tea ceremonies are the most well-known and those who participate in them consider it a time of day for spiritual awareness and reconnecting to inner peace. Although these are elaborate ceremonies, which require instruction, you can create your own simple process. Whether it is your quest for inner peace, or simply to tide you over to dinner and help you keep your intention for nutritional balance and resist overeating at dinner. So, this is could be a comforting, as well as balancing, activity for you.

Of course, the main performer in teatime is the tea and its preparation. Take a hint from the Japanese and have special utensils just for teatime. Even if you have a hectic office schedule, you can keep a special cup or mug, containers with your choice of tea and snack, in a designated space. This could be a simple but distinctive part of your office space. It is there to remind you to appreciate yourself as the day comes to an end. It could be the one process of your day that you look forward to with joy.

Since you will mostly be having teatime alone, you can stock up on your favorite tea. Start by searching the aisle of your favorite grocery and specialty food stores to get familiar with what is available. You will find that there are a variety of choices for you. There is regular tea, which naturally contains caffeine, and decaffeinated tea. There is natural herb tea, most of which will be naturally caffeine-free. There will also be medicinal tea, such as the popular Echinacea that is taken as an immune booster. Pick some of your favorite flavors and start tantalizing your taste buds. A favorite of mine is Earl Grey tea. This tea has the essence of bergamot, a plant in the citrus family. I carry single tea packets of tea in my purse so at 4 o'clock on any given afternoon I usually have a date with a guy named Earl. By drinking one or two cups of black or green tea each day you get natural antioxidants that protect your cells from free radical damage.

Most of the ongoing scientific studies have suggested that even one cup of tea a day can help protect your heart, skin, digestive tract and breasts from free radicals that damage cells and promote disease. You get the best benefit if tea is taken without sugar, artificial sweeteners or cream. So it is rewarding to experiment with natural flavors until you find a tea that is satisfying enough for you to look forward to drinking every day. To make tea, start with cold filtered tap water or bottled water. Heat the water until it is steaming hot and little bubbles start to appear. Do not let the water come to a rolling boil. Measure tea and add to a teapot. Pour water into the teapot with the tea, cover and let steep according to the instructions on the packet. Brewing time is usually one to five minutes; however some medicinal teas take as long as fifteen minutes. Store your tea in an opaque metal, glass or ceramic container instead of plastic. Keep the tea away from heat, light and moisture and it will maintain its flavor. It is not necessary to refrigerate or freeze tea.

To accompany your tea, you can have some of the suggestions in this chapter. If you have tea at your workplace away from home, it is a good thing to carry small containers with fresh or dried fruit, nuts and small sandwiches made with whole grain or multi-grain bread.

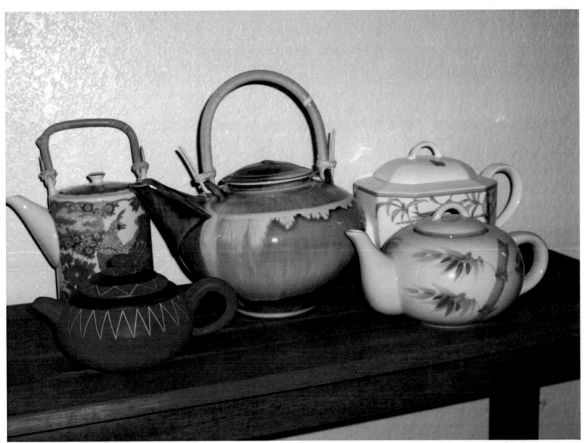

Figure 7 - Teapot Collection

Almond Scones

A scone is the British term for a very flaky biscuit. This scone recipe uses almond meal and currants to add sweetness and increase fiber. This scone could be served with preserves or fruit butter. Some scones can be prepared with cheese, bran or oatmeal and can be served with meat and fish like smoked salmon or cocktail shrimp spread. Scones are rich in saturated fat, coming from the butter, but there is really no substitute if you want a nice flaky scone. Make them bite-size and freeze them so they last for many more teatimes. In any case, this is not a full meal and your body actually needs a small amount of saturated fat daily.

Ingredients

Currant Scones
½ cup almond meal
1 ½ cups pre-sifted flour, with pinches of salt and baking powder
6 tbs. unsalted cold butter
¼ cup sugar
6 oz. currants
1 tsp. pure almond extract
3/4 cup cold low-fat milk
½ tsp. grated nutmeg
1 small beaten egg

Steps

↶Preheat oven to 375 degrees F. In a large bowl mix flour and almond meal. Add sugar, currants and spice. Mix well. Using two knives, cut butter into flour mixture while butter is still cold. The mixture should be like large breadcrumbs or small peas.

↶Mix the extract and milk in a separate container. Add milk mixture to flour until it is just mixed. Do not over mix. This will cause the scones to be tough instead of flaky.

↶Turn on to a floured board and knead very slightly.

↶Flatten dough about ½-inch thick and cut into 1-inch squares or rounds with a cutter.

↶Place on a greased baking sheet and brush with beaten egg.

↶Bake at 375 degrees F for 15-17 minutes until scones are golden brown.

↶Note: Keep all ingredients as cold as possible and the scones will be crispy and flaky.

Black-eyed Pea Hummus

This rich paste is usually made with chickpeas. However, black-eyed peas blend up smooth and tasty. Like chickpeas, they are high in fiber, which is great for keeping your colon young. This is an excellent snack for people who need to balance blood sugar and really good news for those looking for more fiber. It beats drinking those tasteless high-fiber drinks. The tahini or sesame seed butter is rich in calcium, making this a rich and very beneficial anti-aging snack. Tahini, which originated in the Middle East, is now found in serving buckets in health food stores, and in jars in some supermarkets. Spread hummus on sourdough bread or on small triangles of toasted pita bread garnished with sliced tomatoes or roasted red or yellow peppers strips seasoned with herbs such as basil or oregano. Hummus can also be served on a bed of spring greens topped with a crab cake as an appetizer for a celebration meal.

Ingredients

1 cup canned black-eyed peas, rinsed
¼ cup tahini
2 garlic cloves
2 tbs. fresh lemon juice
¼ cup toasted pumpkin seeds
Salt and pepper to taste

Steps

↰———————————————————————————————→

↳Reserve some of the liquid from the can of peas. Save the rest of the peas for salads or soup.

↳Place the peas in a food processor and process until it is crumbly. Add the rest of the ingredients and process until it is smooth. Add some of the pea liquid until it is the consistency of a dip.

↳Transfer to a glass jar and pour olive oil over the top. Refrigerate until time to use.

↳Enjoy as a dip or as a spread.

Cucumber Sandwich

This is a typically British teatime snack, and it is very refreshing. The original is made with white bread with the crust removed. To get the most out of yours, use sourdough white or light multigrain bread. White bread is reported to have a higher glycemic index, which means that it will breakdown into sugar quickly in your body and might increase your blood sugar levels. The good news, though, is that cucumbers are high in fiber, a food characteristic we all need as we age. Use seedless English cucumbers, also called hothouse cucumbers. Cucumbers can actually keep you cool because their water content is high. Additionally, they have electrolytes potassium and magnesium, which helps with blood pressure problems. You can add thin slices of smoked salmon and this will add protein to the sandwich.

Ingredients

1 English cucumber, thinly sliced
Salt and pepper
Thinly sliced tomatoes
Butter
Onion powder

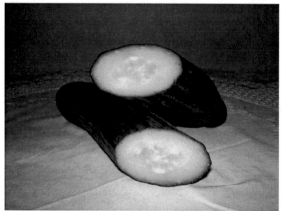
Figure 8- English cucumber

Steps

⟵————————————————————————⟶

↳Cut the crust off sliced bread. Spread with butter.

↳Arrange cucumber on one slice, top with tomato, sprinkle with salt, pepper and onion powder. Cover with other buttered slice.

↳Cut sandwich into small triangles or squares.

↳Place in a container, cover with a damp napkin until read to serve.

Guacamole

Eating this tasty avocado snack often is one of the best things that you can do to slow aging. Avocados have been cultivated since 8000 B.C. I grew up eating the large variety of avocados that weigh almost a pound. This recipe uses the Haas variety grown mostly in California and available in grocery stores all over America. This fruit has real anti-aging punch. It is high in essential fatty acids, which is excellent for aging skin, and it is rich in folate, a body chemical, which helps to regulate your red blood cell count and energy level. Plus, avocados naturally have minerals and vitamins that stabilize blood sugar and support heart health. Ongoing research is giving promising results for people with in high blood cholesterol. So enjoy this every chance you get when they are plentiful in the supermarket.

Ingredients

2 ripe California avocados
1 garlic clove, minced
1 tbs. minced onion
1 small tomato, peeled, seeded and finely chopped
1 tbs. finely chopped cilantro leaves, or roll the leaves and snip with a kitchen scissors
1 tbs. lime juice
¼ tsp. salt and pepper to taste

Steps

⟵⟶

↳ **Cut the avocado in half. Remove the seed and make lengthwise and crosswise cuts in the flesh, then remove the flesh from the skin and place into a serving bowl.**

↳ **Coarsely mash the avocado, and then fold in the rest of the ingredients.**

↳ **Serve with toasted corn chips that are made without preservatives.**

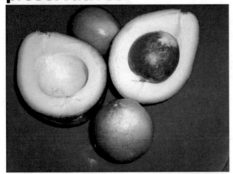

Figure 9 - Freshly Cut Avocado

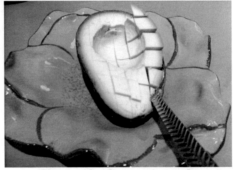

Figure 10 - Cut-up Avocado

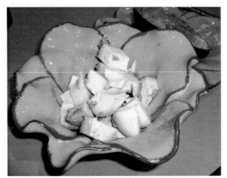

Figure 11 -Diced Avocado

Parsley Pesto

Making pesto is using herbs to their ultimate advantage. Parsley is very rich in vitamin C, and pesto moves it up from being just a piece of garnish on a main course, to being a full-fledged power snack, or cooking sauce. This pesto or herb sauce can be made with basil or even a mixture of cilantro and spinach leaves. Sun-dried tomatoes also make a great pesto. It is thick enough to spread and so can be used on crusty breads or whole grain crackers. It is very flavorful, so it can be used sparingly and will still add a lot of pleasure to snack time. Since a pesto is really a sauce, use it to coat spaghetti or stir it into hot cooked rice. This pesto can also be stirred into vinegar and oil dressing.

Serve on toasted pita bread or crackers with small pieces of grilled meat, chicken or salmon as a snack.

Ingredients

2 cups closely packed fresh parsley leaves
3 garlic cloves
2 tbs. Pine nuts, pecans or walnuts
2 tsp. lemon juice
¼ cup finely grated parmesan cheese
½ tsp. salt
5 tbs. extra virgin olive oil
Dash of hot sauce, water or chicken stock for smooth blending

Steps

⟵⟶

↳**Place the parsley, garlic, lemon juice, and salt in the bowl of a food processor.**
↳**Process until pureed.**
↳**Add 2 tbs. oil, nuts and cheese and continue to puree.**
↳**Transfer to a glass jar.**
↳**Cover top with remaining olive oil.**
↳**Refrigerate in the coldest part of the refrigerator.**

Peanut Sauce

This is a great dip to serve with vegetables like carrots, celery, Napa cabbage leaves and meats like grilled chicken tenders. A salute to Asian origins for introducing us to this wonderful recipe! It moves us beyond the original peanut butter and jelly sandwich and still keeps us in the peanut butter comfort zone. Although some of the ingredients, like Asian five-spice powder, might not be familiar, they are readily available in most supermarkets or your local Asian store. Welcome the great fat in coconut milk. It contains lauric acid a substance that supports both brain and bone health. Coconut milk is reported to help control diabetes, as well as support immune function. Most of the seasonings keep for quite a while in the refrigerator and you can use them in other recipes. I had this at teatime at a resort hotel restaurant served with tiny chicken kebabs, and I was immediately inspired. This tasty snack is definitely active in supporting you against premature aging.

Ingredients

| ¼ cup fresh peanut butter |
| 1/3 cup unsweetened coconut milk |
| 1 tsp. balsamic vinegar |
| ½ tsp. lemon pepper |
| ½-inch piece fresh ginger |
| 1 tsp. honey |
| 1 tsp. Pickapeppa sauce |
| ¼ tsp. Asian five-spice powder |
| ½ tsp. garlic powder |
| Hot pepper sauce and salt to taste |

Steps

↪ Since this recipe is for a small amount, it is better to use a large plastic cup and an electric hand blender.

↪ Place all ingredients in a 16 oz. plastic container; blend with a hand blender until mixture is smooth. Store it in a glass container in the refrigerator.

↪ Serve with sliced green apples, carrots, celery, shredded Chinese cabbage, or any crunchy vegetable of your choice, or even small pieces of grilled chicken tenders or shrimp on skewers.

Salsa

Salsa is a word for sauce. Usually salsa is served in Mexican restaurants as complimentary dips for corn chips and sliced crunchy vegetables like raw jicama. This salsa is convenient and easy to make with a food processor or blender. It is also versatile. Use this as a base and add other fruit like mango or papaya to create mango salsa or papaya salsa. Mangoes and papayas are highly alkaline-forming foods and will keep your blood Hydrogen Ion concentration balanced. This can keep you disease free as you age.

Ingredients

1 can of Mexican-style tomatoes
1 large jalapeno pepper
¼ cup cilantro leaves
Juice of ½ large lime
¼ tsp. salt

Steps

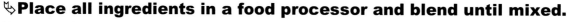

✏ Place all ingredients in a food processor and blend until mixed.
✏ Store in a glass jar in the refrigerator for 1 week.

Toast and strawberries

This snack is very pure and simple. It is a way to enjoy the berry season at its fullest and get the most value. The objective here is to grab the freshness and savor all the enzymes of the fruit, and not destroy the vitamin C and other heat-sensitive phytonutrients by cooking the berries.

Ingredients

2 slices good quality whole grain bread, toasted
6 large strawberries
½ tsp. fructose or table sugar
1 pat of butter

Steps

⟵⟶

🖎Slice strawberries thinly and sprinkle with sugar to bring out the full flavor of the berries. Let stand at room temperature for 5-10 minutes.

🖎Butter the hot toast and place the sliced strawberries on top of both slices.

🖎Serve open-face. The toast can be cut into small snack size pieces.

🖎Serves two.

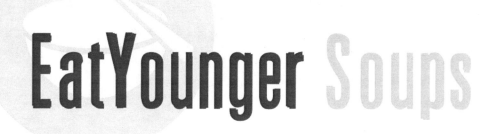

Soups

Introduction to Soups

Soups are comforting and as easy to make as boiling water. This is your chance to choose what nutrients you want for your body at the time and dump it into a stockpot of water and voila! You have soup, effortlessly.

There are recipes for fish stock and vegetable stock. With fish stock you can use your imagination and make any kind of fish soup you desire.

The vegetable stock is great for when you want to try a vegetarian diet or you want to rest your digestive system from processing too much animal protein.

You will like the versatility of soup. It can be a great starter, like the French Onion soup, or make a great lunch or even a main course for dinner. Mostly, these soups give you minerals, vitamins and balanced food combinations that will keep you looking younger and in great shape. Along with this, you will resist illnesses that come with poor food choices. Soup also helps to maintain a healthy weight.

Soups take time, but not your own. Your soup can be cooking and you can be doing countless other things while it just simmers away. You don't have to tend to it after you have it to the point of simmering. Once you have stock, some soups can be made in 10 to 15 minutes, just long enough for the vegetables of your choice to cook. The one soup you will have to attend to is French Onion, but then the French have a love affair with food, so I picked this as the one soup that could raise your passion about being close to the food as it cooks. The end result, and smelling the caramelized onions, is worth it.

It is becoming fashionable to go on soup diets to lose weight. This could be a good habit to retain after you have achieved your goal. Of course, choice of ingredients is very important. Soups made from ingredients that are high in vitamin and mineral content would be superior to ones made with cream and high-starch vegetables, like cream of potato soup. You get lots of soluble fiber from bean and pea soups, and good oils and B vitamins from the avocado soup. So go ahead, think about what you want to achieve and get in the habit of having soup on the menu two or three time a week.

Asian Spice Pea Soup

Baby bok choy is really the star of this pea soup. For starters, it has what you want for aging, phytonutrients like beta carotene and lutein to keep aging eyes healthy. This is a very refreshing broth with the Asian flavors of ginger and star anise. You can make this soup when you want to rest your stomach and yet get some fiber. The ginger would also have a calming effect on your digestion. To add protein, add strips of cooked chicken breast or pork.

Ingredients

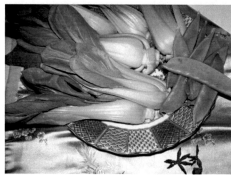

Figure 12 - Baby Bok Choy

2 cup water or vegetable stock
2 green onions, chopped
1 ½-inch piece fresh ginger root, peeled and sliced into thin strips
1 tsp. Asian five-spice powder
½ tsp. each of onion and garlic powder
2 tsp. light soy sauce
1 star anise (optional)
½ tsp. crushed black peppercorns
1 bunch of baby bok choy
2 oz. snow peas, stemmed, stringed, and cut julienne style (into thin strips)
½ cup frozen green peas
1 tsp. toasted sesame oil

Steps

↔

↳ **Rinse the bok choy in water. Cut off the base from bok choy. Separate the leaves, pat dry and coarsely chop.**

↳ **In a saucepan combine the water, green onion, ginger, soy sauce and peppercorns.**

↳ **Simmer until the ginger gives up its flavor, about 10 minutes.**

↳ **Add the five-spice powder, onion and garlic powder, frozen peas, snow peas and bok choy, and cook another 2 minutes.**

↳ **Adjust the seasoning, add the sesame oil, and remove the star anise if used.**

↳ **This recipe serves two.**

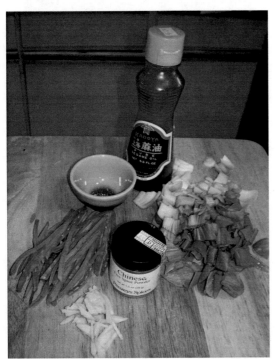

Figure 13 - Ingredients for Asian Spice Pea Soup

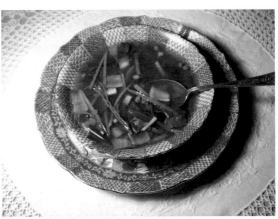

Figure 14 - Asian Spice Pea Soup

Avocado Soup

Avocados bring you so much for so little. This is a cold soup that is the ultimate 'eat yourself younger' food. Avocados have glutathione, a master antioxidant that is involved in protecting your brain cells from damage by free radicals. They contain nutrients that stabilize blood sugar. So this soup helps if you have imbalances in the form of hypo or hyperglycemia. Also present are vitamins and good fats that help to balance cholesterol levels. Indian tribes use the avocado as a condiment, and it is known as Indian Butter. When I was a child, there was an avocado tree in my yard. When it was in season I had avocado, hops bread and butter many mornings for breakfast. I still do this, but now to prevent aging, I use sunflower seed whole wheat bread, but I nix the butter since I would be getting beneficial fat from the avocado. The smoothness of the avocado and crunch of the seeded bread is great for starting your day, and the oils in the fruit helps to keep wrinkles away. The fresh cilantro in this recipe can be kept in a glass of water, covered with plastic in the fridge for about one week.

Ingredients

1 small California avocado
2 green onions
2 tbs. cilantro leaves
½ cup plain non-fat yogurt
½ cup soy milk
½ cup of vegetable or chicken stock
Hot sauce and salt to taste
Dress up this soup with pesticide-free, non toxic flowers, chopped green onions or cilantro for garnish

Steps

↳Cut avocado in half; remove seed and scoop out flesh.

↳Place avocado and other ingredients in a high quality blender.

↳Blend until smooth for about 15 seconds.

↳Taste and add more stock to adjust thickness. Adjust seasonings.

↳Serve cold.

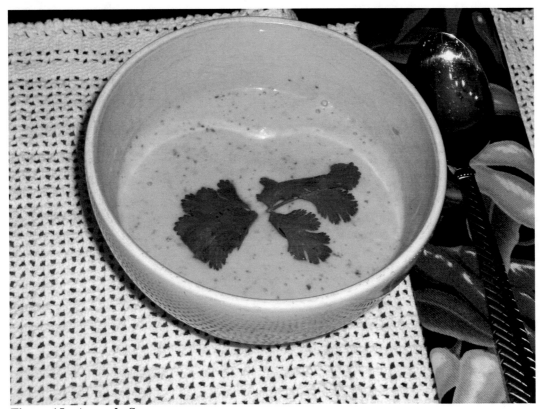

Figure 15 - Avocado Soup

Callaloo

This is one of the national dishes of my birthplace, Trinidad and Tobago. It can be served as soup or as a side vegetable. Traditionally it is made from Taro or dasheen leaves. But it tastes just as good with spinach or green Swiss chard leaves. It is loaded with minerals like iron, and it tastes so good you will want to have 2 or 3 servings of your 5-11 suggested daily requirements of vegetables for Americans. The coconut milk also adds richness along with immune and diabetic support. Whole blue crabs, crab meat or claws are usually added to this soup.

Ingredients

1 bunch of fresh spinach or Swiss chard leaves
8 okra, trimmed and coarsely chopped into 1-inch pieces
4 green onions
½ green pepper
1 sprig fresh thyme or ½ tsp. dried
1 bay leaf
½ cup coconut milk
2 cups chicken stock or salted water
Hot sauce to taste and 1 tsp. Pickapeppa sauce (optional)
2 tsp. ghee or butter
4 oz. crab meat of your choice

Steps

↬Wash and strip the leaves from the greens and cook in a microwave for 2 to 3 minutes until tender, or steam in a stovetop steamer for 5 minutes until tender.

↬Cook the okra, green onion, thyme, and bay leaf with the stock in a covered saucepan over medium heat until the okra seeds turn pinkish, about 15-20 minutes.

↬Add the coconut milk and hot sauce, taste and adjust the seasonings and mix in the cooked greens and simmer for 2 to 3 minutes.

↬Put the hot mixture in a food processor; add the butter or ghee, and pulse to gently blend but not puree the mixture.

↬Pour into a serving dish, add the cooked crab and serve hot.

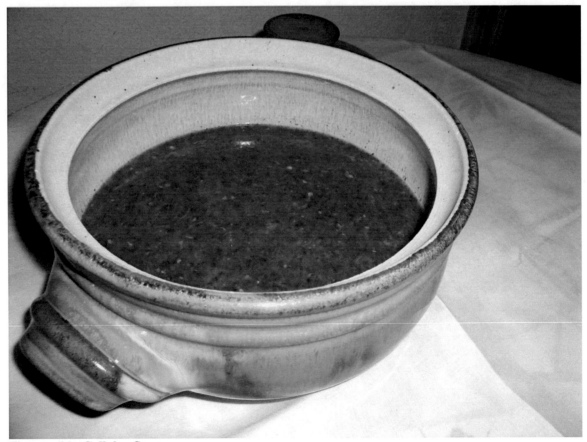

Figure - 16 - Callaloo Soup

Caribbean Three-Bean Soup

Chef Pat Voris wrote this recipe for the <u>Two Billion Dollar</u> <u>Cookbook</u>. I added Green Seasoning, an herb seasoning made by Caribbean cooks and used to season almost any meat, fish or vegetable. It keeps well in the refrigerator for 3 to 4 weeks. (See recipe in Sauce section pg 175). You can also use canned beans and extra virgin olive oil instead of butter. This is a high protein vegetarian meal. Serve it with corn bread. (There is a recipe for cornbread in the breakfast chapter of this book, pg.49).

Ingredients

2 tbs. butter
1 cup chopped yellow onion
1 carrot, peeled and chopped
1 rib of celery, chopped
3 cloves garlic, minced
1 tsp. dried thyme
2 bay leaves
4 cups chicken stock
½ cup red kidney beans, ½ cup pinto beans and ½ cup black beans soaked overnight
1 tbs. olive oil
Salt and pepper to taste, plus 1 tbs. Trinidad green seasoning (see contents)
1 sweet red pepper and 1 green pepper, seeded and diced

Steps

↔

✍Heat butter or olive oil in a large saucepan. Add onions, carrot celery and garlic; cook covered over low heat until vegetables are tender and light colored, about 10 minutes.

✍Add thyme, bay leaves and pour in the stock.

✍Drain and rinse the beans and stir them into the pot. Bring to a boil; reduce heat and simmer partially covered until beans are very tender, about 1 hour.

✍Pour the soup through a strainer, reserving the stock. Discard the bay leaves and transfer ¼ of the solids to the bowl of a food processor fitted with a steed blade. Add 1 cup of the cooking stock if using the processor and process until smooth.

✍Return pureed soup to the pot and stir in additional cooking liquid, 2 or 3 cups, until the soup is of desired consistency.

✍Sauté the peppers in olive oil over low heat, until tender but still crunchy, about 10 minutes.

✍Add green seasoning to peppers and cook until heated. Transfer peppers to soup with a slotted spoon. Taste and adjust salt and pepper. Simmer 10 minutes. Season to taste.

Chili with Beans

I have been told that no self-respecting Texan would eat chili with beans. I am just a "Welcome to Texas" Texan and beans are so good, with their high fiber and protein content that the idea of chili with beans appeals to me. Some grocery stores now carry chili-style beans, green Mexican sauce and chili-style tomatoes that can add even more flavor to your dish. Along with their great taste, beans can balance your blood sugar and lower blood fat as well as give you added B vitamins. Plus, this dish is inexpensive and hearty. Perfecting a chili recipe is almost a vocation of mine. You can easily live on this dish for 3 days by changing out the accompaniments. Try chili with rice, chili with corn tortillas and cheese and for the diet conscious, chili with goat cheese and iceberg or romaine lettuce. I use a chili mix called San Antonio chili mix that I get at a local whole food store. Somehow, I feel the mix is more authentic. However, chili powders and mixes are readily available in most grocery stores.

Ingredients

½ lb. diced meat such as pork, turkey or beef chuck
1 tbs. canola or grapeseed oil
1 green pepper, seeded and finely chopped
1 onion chopped
2 tbs. chili powder
2 clove garlic crushed
Pepper sauce to your taste
1 can of Mexican or chili-style stewed tomatoes
2 tbs. chili sauce
2 cans red kidney beans, or I can black and kidney beans each
1 cup water or stock to adjust thickness. Some chili aficionados swear by dark beer and 1 tablespoon of unsweetened cocoa powder
½ tsp. sea salt
1 tbs. dried oregano or fresh oregano toasted just before using

Steps

Heat oil and garlic in a medium saucepan, over medium heat for 1 minute, and then add onion and green peppers and sauté, stirring frequently for 3 minutes.

Season the meat with salt and pepper and mix with the vegetables until the meat is brown about 5 minutes.

Slowly add the chili powder to the mixture and stir to mix.

Chop the tomatoes in a food processor, then add with chili sauce and stir well. Add cocao powder if desired. Lower the heat and simmer until thickened.

Add the beans and water or stock and let simmer for another 10 minutes to blend the flavors.

Taste and adjust the salt and pepper. This recipe serves for 2-3 meals.

Chili can be garnished with roasted green pumpkin seeds, diced green onions, white cheese like Monterey Jack, or dried oregano.

Cream of Butternut Squash Soup

Go ahead, buy a butternut squash. I make this soup in 4 minutes with the help of a microwave and a very high-powered blender. This vitamin A rich food is my favorite choice for winter soup. It is naturally high in antioxidants that preserve your eyesight, and along with the ginger can give your immune system a boost and keep it in great shape throughout the winter. I keep butternut squash on my kitchen counter as decoration because I just love the shape of this fruit. You can cut pieces off of a very large squash. Once you cut it, remove the seeds and the remaining uncooked piece will keep in your refrigerator for at least 2 weeks.

Ingredients

1 small butternut squash
½ a small onion
1-inch piece ginger, peeled
¼ tsp. pumpkin pie spice or ground cinnamon
Pinch of garam masala, optional
1 cup chicken or vegetable stock

Steps

↪Cut off the rounded part of the squash with the seeds.

↪Put the remaining part of the squash on a microwave dish and cook covered in the microwave until squash is soft about 4-5 minutes depending on the strength of your oven. Cool enough to handle for peeling.

↪Peel squash and add ½ cup to a blender, along with the remaining ingredients.

↪Process on high until mixture is liquefied about 1 minute.

↪Pour into a soup bowl and heat in the microwave oven to your desired temperature.

↪Garnish with garam masala and serve hot.

↪Serves 1 or 2. Save the rest of the cooked squash for making another bowl of soup.

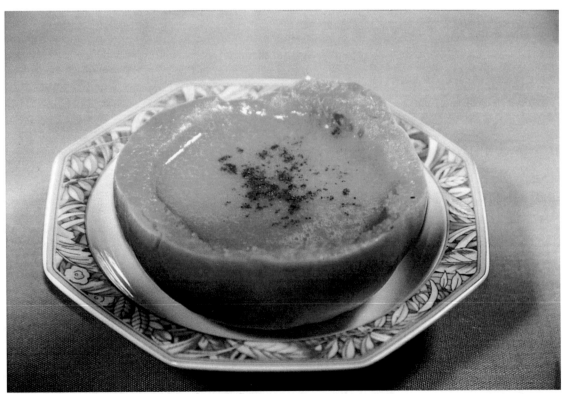

Figure 17 - Cream of Butternut Squash Soup

Lentil Soup

This soup added to your diet will immediately get you on that top list of people through the ages, dating back to the Bronze Age, who appreciated the complexity of high protein and fiber and never worried about obesity. Lentils are an inexpensive and natural form of fiber, folate and magnesium. With this combination in your diet, you can keep your colon youthful and reduce your risk of heart disease, *effortlessly.* Lentils can be adapted to Italian, Indian and fusion cuisine. Just choose your favorite spice and make your soup. It will fill you up, digest slowly and make your day because you will not be craving anything before your next meal or snack. Lentils will keep for 6 months in a jar in a cool, dry place. They come in several varieties, ranging in color from brown to bright orange red. I grew up with the familiar taste of brown lentils, so this recipe has brown lentils. This recipe has Italian herb seasoning but you can substitute one-half teaspoon of dried rosemary and thyme each.

Ingredients

½ cup dried brown lentils
1 carrot, peeled and diced
½ onion, finely chopped
1 tbs. Italian Seasoning or spicy spaghetti seasoning
3 cups water or chicken stock
½ cup good white wine
1 tbs. extra virgin olive oil
1 clove garlic, peeled and minced
Salt and pepper to taste

Steps

↔

✍Place lentils on a clean surface and pick out the broken peas, then place in a strainer and wash under running water, and set aside.

✍In a saucepan over medium heat, add the olive oil and the minced garlic and cook for 1 minute, then add the onion and carrots and cook until the onions are soft, about 3 minutes.

✍Add the onion mixture, water and lentils to a stockpot, bring to a boil, and then lower the heat to medium and skim the froth from the surface of the soup with a slotted spoon.

✍Add the seasoning and simmer until the peas are soft about 30 minutes to an hour.

✍Taste and adjust seasoning with salt, pepper, and hot sauce of your choice.

Lucian Fish Broth

Fish soup is popular as a midday meal in the Caribbean. I got this recipe from a friend who visits St. Lucia, a Caribbean island, often and became enamored with this street food known as Lucian broth. It is very simple; the main ingredients are fish and green figs, which are green bananas. I use small red potatoes since green figs are not readily available to me. However, if you can get green figs, use them because they are very high in iron and the sugar content is very low. This soup is uncluttered. It gets its flavor from the Green Seasoning which has a combination of herbs. (See Green Seasoning recipe in sauces section of this book pg.175) Make a batch of Green Seasoning so that it will be available when you are ready to make the soup. Use a white fish that will hold up to boiling. Good choices are grouper, mahi-mahi and kingfish.

Ingredients

½ lb. grouper filet sliced into 4 pieces
3 tbs. Green Seasoning
4 small red potatoes
1 medium onion, sliced
1 small coarsely chopped green pepper
3 cups fish broth or water
Juice of one lime or 2 tbs. lime juice
1 tsp. salt and black pepper to taste

Steps

⟵──────────────────────────────────⟶

↳**Wash fish in cold water and pat dry. In a shallow dish, season with salt, pepper and Green Seasoning and marinate for 20 minutes.**

↳**Boil potatoes with onion, green pepper, ½ of the lime juice and salt in a medium stockpot until the potatoes are tender.**

↳**Add the fish and boil over medium heat for 5 to 10 minutes until the fish is no longer translucent.**

↳**Taste the broth and adjust salt, add the remaining lime juice and serve immediately.**

↳**Serves two.**

Split Pea Soup

Make this soup a weekly feature on your menu. It is a tradition to use salted pigtail, chicken and root vegetables like dasheen, yam, cassava and small white sweet potatoes in this soup. Although split peas come in yellow or green, I used yellow peas. This soup has a nice balance of carbohydrates, protein and fiber and can keep kids healthy, skipping and jumping for hours. This is a modified version of my mother's split pea soup. I have taken out most of the starchy carbohydrates but it will give you what you need to slow aging. Ideally, beans are low in fat and high in fiber and have enough protein to keep you feeling full…, but here are the pluses - if you have insulin resistance, split peas can stabilize blood sugar and have isoflavones to lower your risk of breast or prostate cancer, and the fiber helps to prevent digestive disorders like Irritable Bowel Syndrome. This soup can be served as a main meal by adding chicken pieces or shrimp, or it can be pureed and served as a starter soup for a festive meal. Either way it is loaded with flavor and 'feel great' factors.

Ingredients

½ cup dried split peas
½ onion
5 whole cloves
1 green pepper, chopped
1 carrot cut in ½-inch pieces
2 or 3 sprigs of fresh thyme or bouquet garni
1 8 oz. can tomato sauce
1 light skin potato, coarsely chopped
1 cup of diced butternut squash or pumpkin
1 tsp. Pickapeppa sauce
Hot sauce
4 cups of stock or salted water
2 tbs. olive oil and 2 oz. chopped smoked pork chops for down home flavor

Steps

←————————————————————————————→

↳Soak the peas in cold water for at least 2 hours or overnight. This helps release some of the gas in the peas, adds moisture and reduces cooking time.

↳Sauté the chopped smoked pork in the oil in a saucepan over medium heat until the meat is brown. Add the carrots and green pepper and cook for 2 to 3 minutes.

↳Drain and rinse the peas and add to a stockpot. Add the water or stock, tomato sauce and the sautéed vegetable mixture, potatoes and pumpkin.

↳Stick the whole cloves into the onion and add to the stockpot along with the thyme or bouquet garni. Bring to a boil, lower the heat and simmer uncovered until the peas are tender, about 2 hours.

↳Taste and adjust salt and pepper and add Pickapeppa sauce. If desired, add chopped greens of your choice and cook until they are done.

↳Serve hot.

Chicken Stock

This is a great soup base, which can also be used for gravies and sauces. Do not restrict yourself to using only chicken. Use any poultry available such as turkey, Cornish hens and duck. Although the time required for making stock is 2 to 3 hours, after first skimming off the scum it can be left to simmer unattended.

Ingredients

Backs, wings, gizzards and necks from 2 chickens
2 quarts cold water
2 carrots cut in 3-inch lengths
2 celery stalks, cut into 3-inch lengths
½ large onion with 6 whole cloves stuck into the surface
2 green onions
3 unpeeled garlic cloves
2 to 3 sprigs of fresh herbs like thyme, rosemary and parsley
2 bay leaves
½ tsp. black peppercorns, or I jalapeno pepper
Salt to taste

Steps

↰Rub the bones with ½ of a lime, squeezing some of the juice. Then rinse chicken under cold running water.

↰Put in a stockpot with the water. Bring to a boil over medium heat. Using a slotted spoon to skim off the scum or foam that rises to the top.

↰Add the vegetables and herbs. Reduce heat after it boils, cover and simmer for 2 hours.

↰Strain into clean glass jars. Discard bones and vegetables. Refrigerate until cool and the fat has hardened on top. Remove fat, leaving about 1 tsp.

↰Store stock in the freezer until ready to use. It can be stored this way for 6 months. In the refrigerator it will last 4-5 days.

Fish Stock

It takes about 30 minutes to make fish stock. It is worth your while because it gives fish sauces and soups a wonderful authentic flavor. Save the heads, tails, bones and shells from fish and shrimp. Do not use the bones of oily fish like salmon because the flavor would be too strong.

Ingredients

Shells from ½ lb. of jumbo shrimp
Bones and head from white-flesh fish
1 medium onion, cut into large pieces
2 celery stalks
1 bay leaf
1 medium carrot
3 fresh thyme sprigs or ½ tsp. dried
3 fresh parsley sprigs
3 cloves garlic
1 cup dry white wine
3 cups of water
5 peppercorns
Juice and zest of ½ lime

Steps

↪Place the bones and shells in a large non-reactive stockpot. Add the onion, carrots, celery, lemon juice, and liquid and bring to a boil. Reduce heat to medium and simmer. Remove the scum or froth that collects on the surface as a result of boiling with a slotted spoon. Add the herbs and peppercorn and simmer on low for 20 minutes.

↪Strain the liquid through a colander lined with cheesecloth.

↪Allow the stock to cool.

↪Store in a glass jar in the fridge for 3 days or freeze for as long as 2 – 3 months.

↪Use with any recipe or sauce that requires fish stock

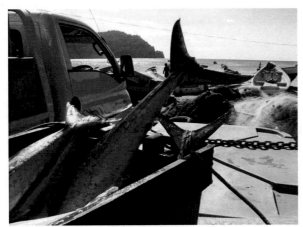

Figure 18 - Fresh Fish Tales – at Las Cuevas Beach, Trinidad, The West Indies

Chicken Tortilla Soup

You can make this soup in a jiffy. I use leftover rotisserie chicken, ready-made salsa or salsa recipe in this book and chicken broth. Add some spices, vegetables and the chips and you are done in about 30 minutes. Don't be fooled by the ease, it is nutrient-dense and balanced for fats and protein.

Ingredients

2 cups of diced Rotisserie chicken meat
½ cup of tomato salsa
1 tbs. canola oil
½ large onion, finely diced
½ green pepper
1 small jalapeno pepper seeded and diced
3 cloves garlic
1 tbs. chili powder
1 tsp. ground cumin
2 yellow squash, coarsely chopped
2 tbs. cilantro, snipped with scissors
¼ cup of corn tortilla chips, about six total
¼ cup grated Mexican Jack cheese
3 cups chicken stock
½ tsp. salt and pepper or hot sauce

Steps

←——————————————————————————————→

↳Use a food processor to chop the onion, garlic and green pepper.

↳ In a medium hot skillet sauté the chopped vegetables until the onion is translucent. ↳Transfer sautéed vegetables to a stock pot.

↳ Add the salsa, chili powder, jalapeno, ground cumin, tortilla chips and the squash.

↳ Add the chicken stock and simmer for 15 minutes.

↳Add the cooked chicken and simmer for 5 minutes.

↳ Add the snipped cilantro and remove from the heat.

↳ To serve: sprinkle with cheese and serve with rice, and sliced avocado.

Vegetable stock

If your recipe calls for stock and you don't want to use a meat-based stock, try boiling vegetables that are in season together. Vegetables like asparagus, broccoli, cabbage and beets might overpower the flavor of others or give your stock an undesired intense color. Stock can be used immediately after being cooled or can be frozen for up to 3 months for future use. You can keep it in the refrigerator for 3-4 days.

Ingredients

2 large onions
5 whole cloves
3 garlic cloves
3 carrots
3 celery stalks
2 bay leaves
Sprig of thyme and rosemary
1 tsp. whole black peppercorns
3 quarts of water
Salt to taste

Steps

↳In a large stockpot, place water and all ingredients except salt. Bring to a boil over medium heat.

↳Skim the surface with a slotted spoon to remove surface scum.

↳Reduce heat to low, cover and simmer for 1-2 hours.

↳Remove from heat, cool and strain into a large container through a colander lined with cheesecloth.

↳Discard vegetables. When stock is completely cooled, refrigerate or freeze for future use.

Chilled Cucumber Soup

Cucumbers have high water content. This is good news if you don't drink your 8 glasses of water. The base of this soup is plain low-fat yogurt. Adopt this soup as a starter to a meal and you will increase your calcium effortlessly. East Indian menus usually include this cold soup. It is known as cucumber Raita. Along with the calcium, natural yogurt has beneficial micro-organisms called probiotics that support good colon health and boost immune function. This soup should always be on your weekly menu if your intent is to eat yourself younger. You will feel good from the inside out.

Ingredients

½ cup plain low fat yogurt
¼ cup of filtered water
¼ cup of finely diced English cucumber
¼ tsp. ground cumin
Dash of pepper sauce or 1 tbs. chopped and seeded green jalapeno pepper
¼ tsp salt

Steps

↳Beat the yogurt with a whisk until smooth.

↳Add the water and stir to combine.

↳Add the cucumber and pepper sauce to the mixture and stir to combine.

↳Sprinkle and stir in the salt and cumin.

↳Cover and chill before serving.

↳ Garnish with cilantro. Refreshing!

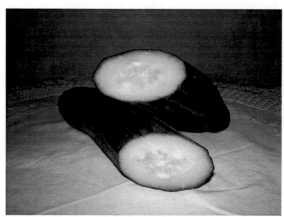

Figure 19 - Seedless Cucumber

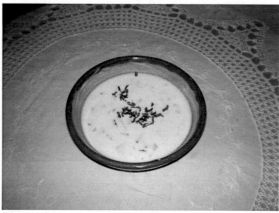

Figure 20 – Chilled Cucumber Soup

EatYounger Salads

Introduction to Salads and Salad Dressings

Salads are a powerhouse of minerals and vitamins to maintain youthfulness. Mostly salads are not cooked, so you get all the nutrients from the fruits or vegetables that your body can absorb. That is, you don't get bogged down into limited choices like iceberg lettuce and tomato or Caesar salad. These are good as fast food fare, but to really take advantage of what a salad has to offer, it is better to use a wide variety of seasonal fruit and vegetables. For instance, you can add a fruit like Kiwi, which has nearly 100% of your daily requirement of vitamin C, to almost any green salad. Vitamin C helps build collagen, a fibrous protein that keeps skin firm. Plus you can effortlessly turn a salad into a balanced meal by adding cooked meat or beans for protein and adding nuts and seeds for balanced amount of good omega oils and vitamin E.

Depending on your choice of ingredients, you get a chance to add soluble and insoluble fiber to your diet. Fiber is the indigestible part of plant matter. It forms bulk for stool, binds to toxins that are eventually released out of the body. Water-soluble fibers found in fresh fruit, vegetables, and beans help your body to keep cholesterol production balanced. Insoluble fibers found in most grains and seeds help your colon to process food quickly and therefore remove toxins and waste out of your body fast. These two functions are good for anti-aging. Choosing different foods gives you a chance to get a variety of necessary benefits and get out of the salad rut.

This book has bean salads, salads with meat and fish, fruit salad like papaya and mandarin, grain salads like quinoa and tabouli, and even a cucumber and tomato and potato salad to keep you in your comfort zone.

One of the most interesting statements I once heard at a nutrition seminar was, "death begins in the colon." I interpreted that to mean that a whole lot of accelerated aging starts from what we choose to put in our mouths. This affects what goes on in our colons and what eventually gets into our blood stream and thus every organ in our body. So go ahead, start a new tradition to have a great salad everyday!

Salad Dressing

There are a few really easy to make salad dressings. In fact, you will only need to have on hand 4 kinds of oil. Extra virgin olive oil for its distinctive flavor and healthy naturalness, canola oil and grape seed oils because they blend so well with different flavors. Grape seed oil is also rich in essential oils that help heal damaged skin and prevent sun damage. Toasted sesame oil is good to add authentic Asian flavor to any dressing. All these oils have essential fatty acids that help you to look and feel younger. The vinegars used in these salads are apple cider vinegar, balsamic and white balsamic vinegar. White balsamic vinegar is like the new kid on the block, but she is very welcome because she adds just the right blend of sweetness and tartness to a salad.

You will find that making dressing is very empowering, because you can control the acidity or the amount and kind of fat that you desire. Also you have the power of knowing exactly what ingredients are in your dressing.

Dressings have an acid ingredient like vinegar or citrus juice, good oil, and salt. You can toss your greens in oil, then add a little citrus or vinegar, taste and sprinkle salt and pepper to your liking. You can also get more creative and add emulsifiers like mustard, yogurt, honey mustard and herbs like basil, chives or garlic. You can make as much or as little as you like.

Of course with all new traditions, your intentions are only wishes if you don't have the right tools to make the change easier. With salads it is best to have a hand blender or food processor for mixing dressings. However, a medium bowl and a whisk will do just as well. To store salad dressing it helps to have small storage bottles with airtight stoppers. Most dressing can keep in the fridge for one or two weeks. The best part is that you can control the ingredients and avoid using dressings that have preservatives for shelf life or other ingredients that you do not desire.

You can choose any of these salads for lunch or for dinner as part of the meal.

For dinner, use a smaller portion if it is part of the meal. Salads with meat or fish can serve as a full meal.

Citrus Dressing

Use this dressing with fruit salads. It will keep the high vitamin C theme going. Use fresh-squeezed juice; the vitamin C content is higher than juice. Expect all your skin problems to clear up and just be radiant since this salad is going to help you build more collagen, a key ingredient in healthy youthful looking skin.

Ingredients

¼ cup fresh grapefruit juice or citrus of your choice and 1 tbs. zest of the fruit
1 tbs. white balsamic vinegar
1 tbs. water
5 large basil leaves, cut into slivers
5 tbs. canola oil
¼ tsp. salt
½ tsp. freshly ground black pepper
2 tsp. minced peeled ginger

Steps

⟵⟶

↳Use a small bowl and a whisk to mix the grapefruit juice and zest with the balsamic vinegar, water salt and pepper.
↳Add the slivered basil and the ginger. Then let the dressing rest for 5 minutes.
↳Then, slowly, in a drizzle, whisk in the oil.
↳Serve often with any salad greens of your choice.

Green Onion Dressing

This dressing is rich and powerful. The fat is reduced, but the yogurt helps to keep the creaminess and make it rich in calcium and amino acids. You get plenty of food value in this dressing, including essential fatty acids. Use it with any type of salad greens. It will last for a week in your refrigerator. Spicy spaghetti seasoning is available at local grocery stores and stores that sell in bulk.

Ingredients

4 green onions
4 tbs. of fresh cilantro leaves
½ cup plain non-fat yogurt
2 tbs. olive oil
1 tbs. apple cider vinegar
1 tbs. balsamic vinegar
¼ tsp. salt
Dash of hot sauce to taste
1 tbs. spicy Italian seasoning or spicy spaghetti seasoning

Steps

↬Place yogurt first, then all ingredients, in high-powered blender and process for about 10 –12 seconds.

↬Serve on your favorite green salad.

↬Store in a glass jar in the fridge.

Note: Use white balsamic vinegar if you want a light green dressing. Add 1 tsp. honey if the dressing is too tart.

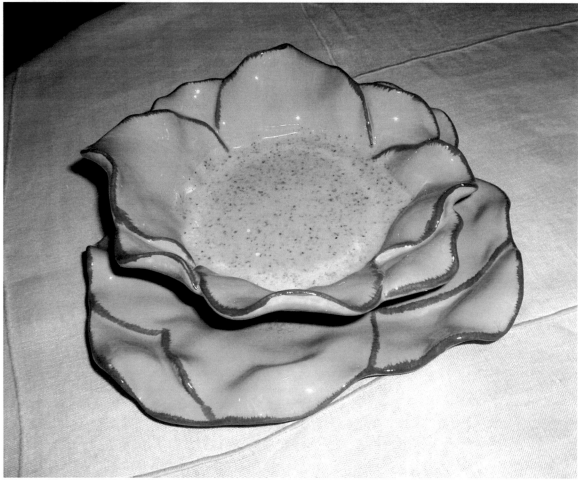

Figure 21 - Green Onion Dressing

Honey Mustard Dressing

Once you master making this dressing, you will want to stop using dressings with preservatives and words that scare you. This little dressing is very natural. Don't be afraid of the oil, it is good for your skin and gives you the immune friendly antioxidant vitamin E. Honey mustard is found in the same section with mustards in most grocery stores. Add 1 more tablespoon of oil if the dressing is too tart.

Ingredients

2 tbs. apple cider vinegar
1 tbs. water
Salt and pepper to taste
1 tbs. honey mustard
4 tbs. olive oil

Steps

↔

↳ Mix vinegar, water, salt, and pepper and, let stand for 5 minutes at room temperature.

↳ Add honey mustard.

↳ Wisk in the olive oil in a dribble until it is emulsified or completely mixed, or use a hand blender.

↳ Serve with salad of your choice.

Sesame Seed Vinaigrette

Nothing says Asian flair like toasted sesame seeds. This dressing would add an Asian taste to any salad greens, including the Chinese classics like grated carrots, mixed sprouts and Napa cabbage.

Ingredients

1 tbs. toasted sesame seeds
1 tsp. toasted sesame oil, plus 2 tbs. grape seed oil
2 tbs. freshly-squeezed orange juice
1 tsp. orange zest
1 tsp. soy sauce
1 tbs. white balsamic vinegar or rice wine vinegar
1 tsp. brown sugar

Steps

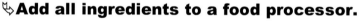

↳Add all ingredients to a food processor.
↳Process to mix thoroughly.
↳Serve over grated carrots, grated cucumbers, and mixed sprouts.

Carrot Salad

This is such a beneficial little salad that you can always have it in your refrigerator. It is filled with fresh antioxidants from the carrots and digestive enzymes from the fresh pineapple. You can eat this salad as a snack when you want something sweet and still stay within your '5 a Day' fruit and vegetable habit. And of course, it makes a great salad served with spring greens.

Ingredients

2 carrots, grated
2 tbs. white raisins
2 tbs. minced fresh or canned crushed pineapple
1 tsp. fresh lime juice or white balsamic vinegar
1 tsp. grape seed oil
Salt and pepper to taste

Steps

↳ Mix all ingredients together in a medium bowl.
↳ Chill.
↳ ENJOY! ☺

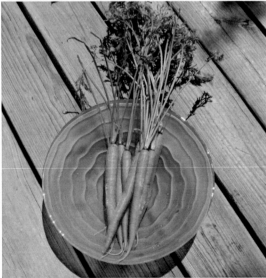

Figure 22 - Fresh Organic Carrots

Black-eyed Pea Salad

A real cholesterol challenger using natural fiber is at play in this recipe. This salad is also known as Texas Caviar and shows up on well-dressed tables all over Texas on New Year's Eve. After the celebration, make this salad using other beans such as a mixture of black and white beans. The theme here is to keep up with fiber and also a good source of non-meat protein, which the peas provide. Protein helps to speed up metabolic processes that rev up your vitality. If you are not used to eating beans, you might experience problems with gas. Digestive enzymes capsules sold in the vitamin section of your grocery store or in health food stores help. Be sure to take enzymes before you start your meal.

Ingredients

16 oz. can cooked black-eyed peas or any other combination of small beans
½ medium onion, chopped
2 cloves garlic
½ red bell pepper, chopped
½ green bell pepper, chopped
½ cucumber peeled, seeded and chopped
3 tbs. minced cilantro leaves
1 jalapeno pepper, seeded and chopped
2 tbs. balsamic vinegar
2 tbs. water
1 tsp. honey mustard
6 tbs. canola oil
¼ tsp. salt
Hot sauce to taste

Steps

↳Drain black-eyed peas in a colander, rinse under cold running water and place in a salad bowl.

↳Add the chopped peppers, onion, cucumber and cilantro to the bowl.

↳In a separate container or blender, add the vinegar, water, honey mustard and salt, mix and then slowly whisk in the canola oil.

↳Add the dressing to the peas or beans mixture. Cover and refrigerate overnight. This salad will last in the refrigerator for one week.

Cilantro Potato Salad

Potatoes are the ultimate comfort food. French fries are on the top of most everyone's list as the choice fast food. I really had to grow up and call in all my willpower to stop eating mashed potatoes as the major "raise my spirit and stay in bliss" food. Potatoes, along with guava and pineapple jam, fed my carbohydrate craving for years, until I discovered that I could change the spices and thereby change the feeling and really get new sensations with this vegetable. This recipe has a southwestern flair, but you can give your potato salad a Mediterranean, Indian or German flavor by changing the spices and dressings. Then your palate and your emotions get a new experience. Potatoes are high in potassium, a mineral that helps resist aging. This recipe also uses low-fat live cultured yogurt in the dressing. This helps to balance the fat and increase the protein and calcium to give increased anti-aging, nutritional support.

Ingredients

5 new potatoes
¼ cup chopped cilantro leaves
1 jalapeno chili
½ green bell pepper, peeled, seeded and chopped
½ medium onion, finely chopped
1 clove garlic, minced
¼ cup plain lowfat yogurt with live cultures
1 tbs. mayonnaise
1 tsp. Dijon mustard
1 tsp. chili powder
Salt and pepper to taste

Steps

↜━━━━━━━━━━━━━━━━━━━━━━━━━━━━━━━━➤

↳Place potatoes in a saucepan and cover with water. Boil over high heat until they are fork tender, about 15 to 20 minutes. Remove from heat, drain and cool.

↳Cut cooled potatoes into 1-inch pieces and set aside in a serving bowl. Add minced onion and green peppers.

↳ Mix yogurt, mayonnaise, mustard, chili powder, cilantro leaves, garlic and a dash of salt and pepper in a small bowl.

↳Add yogurt mixture to potatoes. Toss with a spoon until the yogurt dressing is well mixed with the potatoes.

↳Adjust salt and pepper to taste.

↳Serve cold.

Cinco de Mayo Salad

Adopt this as a great salad for a celebration. But don't save it for May 5th only. Celebrate your life as often as you want with this convenient meal. Put it on your menu for dinner or for lunch. The chicken is so versatile; the dressing is balanced, creamy and rich in calcium, the mineral that keeps a bounce in your step with youthful bones. The seeds are there to rejuvenate your colon on a regular basis. The avocado with its healthy oils and minerals add youth sustaining benefits. You can use whatever seeds you desire, just don't leave them out without adding something that will replace the fiber.

Ingredients

2 chicken breast
1 ½ tsp. toasted and ground cumin seeds
½ tsp. toasted and ground coriander seed
Salt and pepper to taste
1 tsp. garlic powder
1 tsp. onion powder
1 tbs. olive oil
Juice of ½ lemon
½ cup thinly sliced carrots
½ red pepper, peeled and thinly sliced
½ green pepper, peeled and thinly sliced
2 green onions, chopped
3 tbs. finely chopped fresh cilantro leaves
¼ cup plain non-fat yogurt
2 tbs. mayonnaise
2 tbs. lime juice
¼ cup toasted pumpkin seeds
2 avocados, peeled and cut into wedges
Green leaf lettuce leaves and black olives for garnish

Steps

↰Brush the chicken with olive oil, season with coriander, half of the ground cumin, salt and pepper. Grill until chicken is cooked and tender, about 7 minutes on each side. Set aside to cool. Slice the cooled chicken into wedges 2 inches long.

↰Blend yogurt, mayonnaise, lime juice, remaining cumin, cilantro, salt and pepper
in a salad bowl. Add yogurt mixture, chicken, vegetables and cilantro and toss.

↰Serve on a bed of lettuce and garnish with olives, avocado and toasted pumpkin seeds.

↰Serves two.

Green Bean and Sesame Salad

Don't let the familiarity of this vegetable fool you. This supposedly ordinary favorite has powerful 'eat younger' assistance. Although frozen beans are readily available, use fresh green beans when they are abundant in the super or farmer's markets. Green beans have enough protective nutrients like vitamin A and C to support your immune system and protect your cardiovascular system. The beans will keep their green color when steamed or cooked in the microwave. Sesame seeds, with their nutty taste and delicate crunch, are rich in copper and anti-inflammatory minerals that can naturally help with rheumatoid arthritis. With this salad as regular fare, you might just get rid of aging aches and pains.

Ingredients

1 pound fresh green beans
1 tbs. sesame seeds
2 tbs. slivered raw almonds
2 green onions
½ red pepper, cut into thin strips
2 tbs. apple vinegar
¼-inch piece of ginger minced
2 cloves garlic, minced
2 tsp. soy sauce
1 tsp. sugar
3 tbs. canola oil
1 tsp. toasted sesame oil
Salt and pepper to taste

Steps

↺Roast the sesame seeds in a dry hot skillet until brown, about 2 minutes and set aside to cool.

↺Cook the green beans in a microwave oven with 2 tbs. of water in a covered container for 1 to 2 minutes, until they lose their rawness, but are still crisp.

↺Rinse the beans in ice-cold water and drain well.

↺Mix the dressing by placing the vinegar, sugar, soy sauce, minced garlic and ginger in a bowl.

↺Then slowly whisk in the oils. Taste, adjust taste for salt and pepper.

↺Add the beans and seeds to the mixture in the bowl and toss to coat beans.

↺Serve at room temperature.

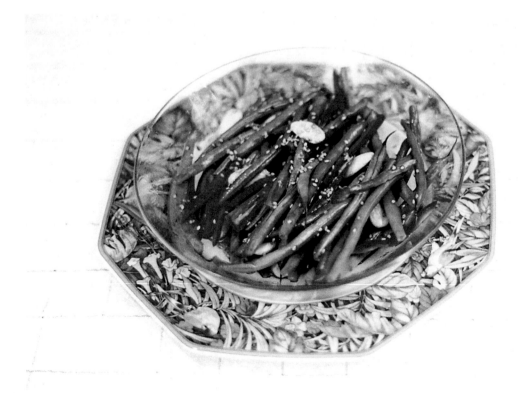

Figure 23 - Green Bean and Sesame Salad

Papaya Mandarin Salad

**Papayas have marvelous enzymes that improve digestion. You will absorb more nutrients from all of the meal. And they also have the capacity to keep your body fluids neutral. This keeps you well and your body performing as if you are younger. Voila! You are eating younger. Pick papayas that are yellow but firm. Overripe papayas will not perform at their top capacity.
Use the finest section of a grater to remove the outermost colored portion of the tangerine rind. This is the zest. It has intense flavored oil of tangerine. The white pith underneath the zest is bitter, so try to avoid it as you remove the zest.**

Ingredients

1 small ripe papaya, diced into bite-size pieces
2 peeled and segmented mandarin oranges or tangerines
Alfalfa sprouts, salad greens and chopped cilantro
¼ cup pistachio nuts
4 very thin slices of Proscuitto or pan-fried bacon for garnish
Juice of 1 mandarin orange
Dressing: 1 tsp. tangerine zest
4 tbs. fresh tangerine juice
2 tsp. apple cider vinegar or lime juice
Sea-salt and white pepper to taste
6 tbs. extra virgin olive oil

Steps

↪Eat this salad with a zesty, freshly-made mandarin dressing. Mix all ingredients in the dressing, except the oil, in the bowl in which the salad is to be served. Slowly whisk in the olive oil. Place the salad ingredients in the bowl with the dressing. Mix in the dressing by tossing with tongs. You are ready to eat.

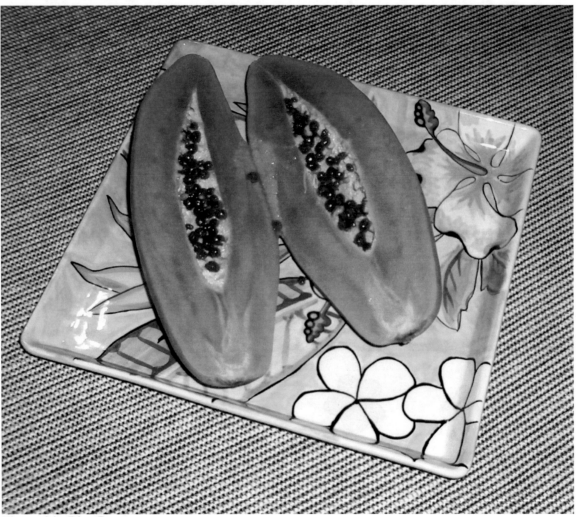

Figure 24 - Ripe Papaya

Vegetable Power Salad

Eat this salad often. It is a great way to get your "5 a day" of green foods; especially if you work 9 to 5 and don't have energy to cook. You must, however, find some time to shop the vegetable aisle of your favorite whole food store. This recipe gives you two to four single servings in a week. One fabulous salad and your have started a new eat younger habit with veggies. No standing in fast food lines with this in the fridge. Add a 3 or 4 oz. piece of turkey or tofu, a slice of multigrain bread, and you are all set for the evening.

Ingredients

2 cups of broccoli, chopped
1 cup of carrots, coarsely chopped
½ cup of yellow squash, diced
1 cup zucchini, diced
1/3 cup sesame or sunflower seeds
½ cup raw almonds
½ cup raisins
4 tbsp. scallions or chives, chopped
2 tbsp. apple cider vinegar
4 tbsp. extra virgin olive oil
1 green leaf lettuce, washed and leaves separated

Steps

↳Steam broccoli and carrots for 2 minutes. If steaming in a microwave oven, cook for 1 minute and remove immediately. The broccoli should turn deep green and stay firm. Cool vegetables to room temperature by putting them in a colander and pouring ice cold water over them. Transfer to a serving bowl.

Toast sesame seeds in a hot skillet for 2 minutes or until seeds begin to pop out of the pan. Let cool.

↳Add raisins and scallions to the serving bowl and stir in lemon juice and olive oil or dressing of choice. Toss with tongs.

↳Serve over lettuce leaves, and garnish with toasted seeds and almonds. Sprinkle with salt and pepper.

↳Serves four. (If it is used as the main meal it serves two.)

Quinoa Salad

This salad is loaded with fiber and vitamins A and E from the berries and nuts. It will help keep both your kidney and colon young. Ancient Inca Indians got their protein from quinoa and even named it the "mother grain." Along with the eight essential amino acids in its protein, it is also loaded with iron, potassium, zinc and calcium. One cup of quinoa has as much calcium as a quart of milk. You will like the nutty texture and flavor of this grain. It cooks in 20 minutes just like rice, so go ahead and use it like rice in main menus. Pronounce it 'keen wa" when you ask for it at your local health food grocery store. This salad is especially beneficial if you are trying to get more protein from a source other than meat.

Ingredients

½ cup of quinoa, rinsed well and drained
1 cup of water
4 green onions, finely sliced
¼ cup dried cranberries
3 tbs. cilantro leaves, chopped
1 stalk celery, chopped
¼ cup toasted chopped pecans
3 tbs. extra virgin olive oil
1 tbs. lemon juice
1 tbs. white balsamic vinegar
1 tsp. honey mustard
Pinch of salt
Black pepper
8 lettuce leaves, 2 large tomatoes and cucumber slices for garnish

Steps

↪Add quinoa to water; bring to a boil on the stove or in your microwave. Then cover and cook for 15 minutes on low, microwave at 50% power. Let stand until water is absorbed and quinoa is cooked. Cool to room temperature.

↪In a large salad bowl add the vinegar and lemon juice, mustard, salt and pepper then slowly whisk in the olive oil.

↪Add the cooled quinoa and other ingredients to the bowl and mix then with salad tongs.

↪Present this salad on a large plate covered with lettuce leaves, and line the rim with thinly sliced tomatoes and cucumbers. Remove the salad from the bowl and place in the center of the plate.

↪Let stand at room temperature for 1 hour.

↪Serve at room temperature.

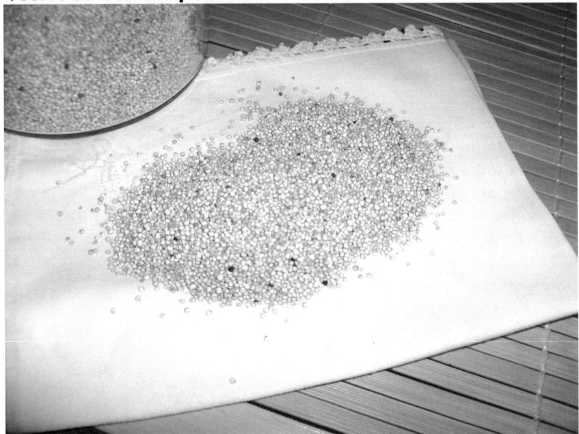

Figure 25 - Uncooked Quinoa grains

Shrimp and Artichoke Salad

This combination says love yourself all over. Who is looking for the elusive element, chromium? If you are diabetic, or have a genetic link from one of your parents, you should be! Chromium helps to regulate blood sugar. Artichokes can supply about 10% of your daily requirement of chromium along with potassium and magnesium. Celebrate your life often with this salad. Make the dressing first and refrigerate it. You can assemble the salad on individual plates when you are ready to serve. Then add the dressing. Artichokes can be found in cans or jars. Discard the liquid and rinse to reduce the tartness.

Ingredients

1 garlic clove
1/8 tsp. salt
1 tbs. apple cider vinegar
1 tbs. water
1 tsp. honey mustard
Pepper to taste
3 tbs. olive oil
3 tbs. julienne basil leaves
½ small red onion, finely sliced
½ pound of cooked and peeled large shrimp
1 6 oz. jar of quartered artichoke hearts or 6 oz. cooked frozen artichokes
1 Boston bib lettuce head
Black olives for garnish

Steps

↳Dice the garlic with salt and mash it to a pulp.

↳In a small bowl mix the garlic and mustard. Add the vinegar and water and let stand for 5 minutes.

↳Slowly whisk in the olive oil until it is a creamy dressing.

↳Season with pepper and more salt to your taste.

↳Add the basil and onions and refrigerate the dressing.

↳Drain the bottle of artichoke hearts, cut them into quarters, add to the shrimp and then place mixture on a bed of lettuce.

↳Add the dressing and enjoy.

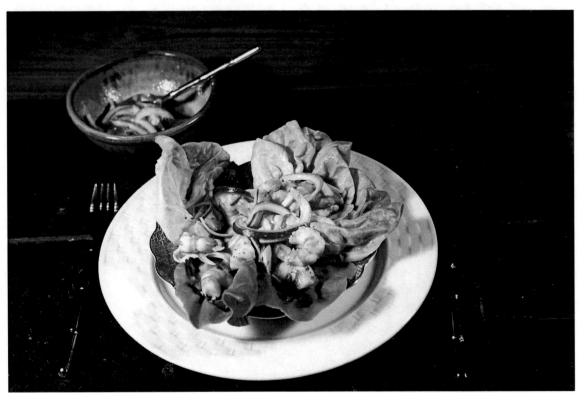

Figure 26 - Shrimp and Artichoke Salad

Southwestern Corn Salad

This is a very colorful dish that tastes great and is loaded with good qualities. The onions help to increase the breakdown of fat in the meal and get it out of your body before it has time to settle on your hips and belly. Cabbage is a cruciferous vegetable that helps guard you against cancer and keeps your colon in a youthful state.

Ingredients

Kernels removed from 2 ears of cooked corn, about 1 cup of kernels
1 cup of grated or finely sliced red cabbage
¼ medium onion, thinly sliced
1 tsp. capers
2 tbs. finely chopped fresh parsley or cilantro
1 tsp. apple cider vinegar or fresh lime juice
1 tsp. white balsamic vinegar
1 tsp. water
2 tsp. honey Dijon mustard
1 tsp. toasted, ground cumin seeds
Pinch of salt and pepper
3 tbs. olive oil

Steps

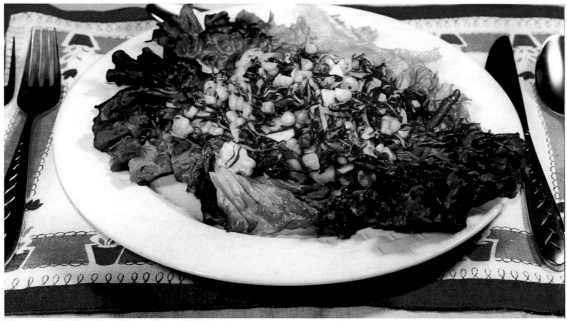

↳Mix and toss cabbage, corn, onion, capers and parsley.
In a small dry skillet, toast cumin seeds over high heat for 1
minute, transfer to a mortar and pestle and grind to release the
flavor.

↳Make vinaigrette by combining vinegars, water, mustard and
cumin. Add salt and pepper to taste.

↳Set aside for 5 minutes.

↳Slowly whisk in oil.

↳Pour over salad and toss.

↳Place on a bed of green leaf lettuce and serve on individual
plates.

↳Serves two.

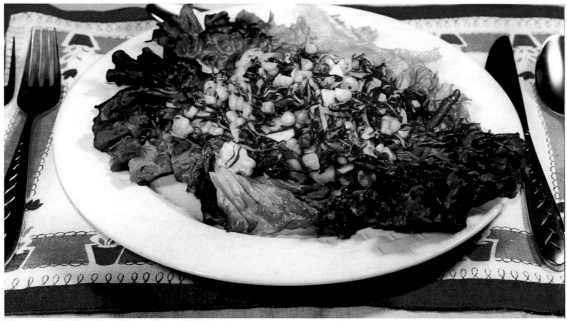

Figure 27 - Southwestern Corn Salad

Baby Spinach and Arugula with Strawberry Dressing

Make this salad often in the spring when strawberries are fresh and you want to hold on to that young, fleeting feeling of renewal and the rebirth of freshness. The vitamin C in the salad is at paramount proportions; it is everywhere in the greens, the berries, the juice, and it will show up as more collagen in your skin. Seize the dish!

Ingredients

3 cups of fresh baby spinach leaves
1 cup arugula leaves
1 pint of fresh organic strawberries, sliced
1/3 cup pecans or walnut pieces
Dressing:
¼ cup fresh-squeezed orange juice
10 organic strawberries pureed with 1 tsp. sugar and 1 tbs. water
1 tbs. fresh lemon juice or 1 tbs. white balsamic vinegar
3 tbs. canola oil
Dash of hot sauce
1/8 tsp. salt
Crumbled goat cheese and alfalfa sprouts as garnish

Steps

☞To make the dressing, place the 10 strawberries, water, and sugar in a blender and puree until liquid. Add the orange juice, lemon juice or vinegar and salt and blend until smooth and has a creamy consistency. Let stand for 5 minutes.

☞Slowly add oil with blender running until oil is well mixed. Add pepper or hot sauce to taste.

☞Pour some dressing into a large bowl.

☞Add spinach, strawberries and nuts.

☞Toss with salad tongs until leaves are covered with dressing.

☞Serve with crumbled goat cheese or grated white cheese of your choice.

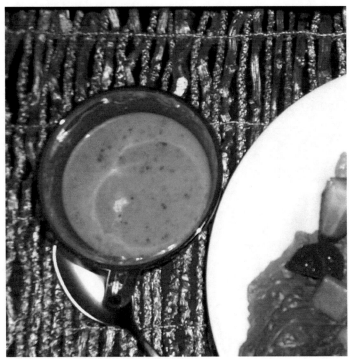

Figure 28 - Strawberry Dressing

Tabouli Salad

I first tasted Tabouli at a Syrian luncheon, and ever since I have been fascinated and hooked by its texture and taste. Its main ingredient is wheat that has already been processed to produce bulgur. To this are added parsley, mint, onions and spices. Fortunately, it is possible to purchase a boxed mix of this salad in a dry form that you can easily re-hydrate by adding the required amount of water. Tabouli is available from most well-stocked grocery stores, as well as from health food stores. This grain salad is worth searching out. It is also called tabouleh. Tabouli will help increase your dietary fiber, and research has revealed that it will help to keep you slender. Increasing your intake of grains keeps the colon clean and helps in absorption of other minerals and vitamins required to delay aging and resist disease. The eggs give added protein and balances out the meal. The peppers and parsley give you vitamin C to support your immune system.

This is good to use either as a side salad on whole lettuce leaves, or for a quick lunch or snack with pita bread.

Ingredients

¼ cup Tabouli mix and ¼ cup of water
½ red bell pepper, finely diced
½ cup, finely diced fresh parsley
½ green bell pepper, finely diced
2 jumbo eggs, boiled and chopped
2 tbs. extra virgin olive oil
Ground black pepper to taste

Steps

↬Place the tabouli mix in a salad bowl. Add the water and let stand at room temperature until the water is completely absorbed, about 20 minutes.

↬Cover the eggs with water and boil for 10 minutes. Discard water and cool in cold water.

↬If desired, peel the peppers with a vegetable peeler and dice.

↬Remove shell from eggs and chop or grate using the large opening on the grater.

↬Add the parsley, peppers and eggs to the salad bowl and mix with the tabouli, chill until ready to serve.

↬Add the olive oil and black pepper when ready to serve.

Warm Broccoli and Asparagus Salad

When you want high-level nutrition and you are serious about resisting cancer, broccoli is your vegetable. The health-giving phytonutrients in this vegetable give hope for the cure for cancer, which I suspect is in direct relationship to how we EAT! Shiitake mushrooms are in here to increase your immune stamina and keep you safe from seasonal colds. This salad can get you safely through the winter without a sniffle and with a youthful smile on your face.

Ingredients

1 bunch broccoli
1 dozen asparagus spears
5 sliced and cooked shiitake mushrooms
2 tbs. extra virgin olive oil
2 tbs. balsamic vinegar
2 tbs. water
2 cloves garlic
½ tsp. salt
¼ tsp. black pepper

Steps

$\longleftarrow$ —————————————————————————————— $\longrightarrow$

↳Remove broccoli florets from stalks and separate into 1 to 1 ½-inch pieces.

↳Cut the tough ends off the asparagus.

↳Place garlic and salt on a chopping board and finely chop with a knife, or use a mortar and pestle.

↳Put the oil in a skillet and heat over medium heat. Add the garlic and salt mixture and heat for one or two minutes. Do not brown.

↳Add the asparagus and broccoli and sauté for one minute. Add the water when the skillet becomes dry and continue to sauté.

↳Add the balsamic vinegar and the cooked shiitake mushrooms.

↳Place the vegetables in a serving dish. Drizzle with oil and toss with tongs to cover. Serve immediately.

Cucumber and Tomato Salad

Bring more harmony, coolness and simplicity to your life with this salad. Because of their high water content, cucumbers are hydrating and satisfying. Serve this salad with butter lettuce or Boston Bibb. Add slices of fresh mozzarella cheese to increase its calcium and protein content. The perfect mate for this salad is a simple vinaigrette dressing.

Ingredients

1 large English cucumber
1 large tomato
2 green onions
Basil leaves
Black Olives

Steps

◁──────────────────────▷

↳Slice cucumber and tomatoes very thin.
↳Arrange on a plate, alternating cucumber and tomato slices in a circle.
↳Place basil leaves and olives in the center.
↳Serve with vinaigrette dressing of your choice.

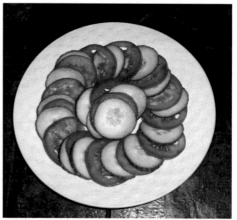

Figure 29 - Cucumber and Tomato Salad

EatYounger Dinner

Dinners

These dinners were chosen so that you can expand your experiences with different foods as you continue to focus on slowing your aging, feeling great and looking good. Some of the food will be a new version of a familiar recipe, like our Crab Burger. It is the anti-aging answer to a hamburger. The crab has less fat, has not been manipulated with hormones, and is easier on your digestive system than beef. This takes eating a hamburger to a higher level and gives you a chance to have more adventure with food.

You might notice that the dinner recipes concentrate primarily on cooking the protein part of the meal. I give suggestions of what vegetables to pair with them, but you can pick and choose any vegetable or salad from this book.

It is extremely important to serve green leafy vegetable like kale, spinach and bok choy, and salads with each meal. There are suggestions in the menu section. It is my philosophy that vegetables should be kept in as pure a form as possible. For this reason, I only steam or microwave vegetables until they are green but crisp, and serve them with a teaspoon of extra virgin olive oil and a squeeze of lime juice, or a dash of black or white balsamic vinegar. Vegetables can be garnished with thinly sliced red or green onions. Try to resist the temptation to cook vegetables in cheese, cream or buttery sauces. This will increase the saturated fat in your diet, and your overall dietary fat can become imbalanced and cause you problems with blood circulation. Most research on food is now showing that the high temperatures used for frying and sautéing in saturated fat causes chemical changes in the fat that is detrimental to the body, and can speed up aging. Plus, by simply steaming the vegetables, you get to enjoy the true nuances in taste and texture of the food and the full benefits of all the minerals and vitamins. Cook fresh or frozen vegetables as close to serving time as possible. This will preserve the nutritional value until it is eaten.

Vegetables and fruits have essential vitamins, minerals and bio-active substances like antioxidants, unique to plants that help us resist aging. For instance, carrots have the antioxidant beta-carotene; tomatoes have lycopene, a free radical scavenger; and corn, kale and spinach have lutein that protects our eyes from aging. That's just the beginning of what is known about plants, but it is enough for me to make a habit of eating my greens.

The U.S. Department of Agriculture (USDA) recommends that the serving size of most cooked leafy vegetables is one-half cup and for salads it is one whole cup. Get in the habit of eating 2 or 3 kinds of vegetables with at least two of your meals so that you get enough of the five to seven recommended standard servings per day. I bet you won't feel hungry with this new habit because vegetables also have fiber, which adds bulk and helps you to feel satisfied longer.

I don't recommend specialty diets like a high-protein diet, but I do feel that you should get adequate amounts of protein. Protein provides essential amino acids, which is necessary to make enzymes that facilitate metabolic events that help resist aging in cells. If you don't get enough protein, you can be constantly missing messages coded at the cellular level that help resist aging. Worse yet, you could be eating too many starchy carbohydrates to make up your daily calories. If you do not use up this carbohydrate fuel exercising two to three hours per day, this can cause accelerated aging and obesity as early as your thirties. This is the philosophy of one of the most insightful doctors on aging, Diana Schwarzbein, M.D., as presented in her book, <u>The Schwarzbein Principle: The truth about losing weight, being healthy and feeling younger.</u>

The USDA recommended serving size for protein is 4 ounces, raw. Most of the recipes in this book will give you about three to four ounces of cooked protein, which might seem like a small amount, but it will get the job done without stressing or overloading your cells. That means you will have what you need to keep you looking and feeling younger.

Caramelized Quail

These little birds are festive and tender, so you can save them for when you are celebrating. They cook quickly and this recipe is designed to get you out of the kitchen with the utmost speed.

Ingredients

½ tsp. rosemary
1 tsp. dried thyme
Juice of 1 lime
Salt and freshly ground pepper
1 tsp. brown sugar
2 tbs. olive oil
4 quail

Steps

←——————————————————————————→

↳Using kitchen shears, cut along the backbones of the quail and remove them. Set the birds, breast side up and press on the breastbones with the heel of your hands to flatten them.

↳Season the quail with lime juice, salt and pepper, and the dried herbs.

↳Set a large iron skillet over high heat. When it is hot, add the brown sugar and stir as it melts and bubbles then add the oil and stir. Do not let the sugar harden. When the sugar and oil is combined, then add the quail, breast side up, lower the heat to medium and cook until they are a dark brown about 1-2 minutes. Turn the quail and cook the other side until the breast skin is crisp and brown. Add small amounts of oil to stop the birds from sticking.

↳Place the quail in an oven heated to 450 degrees F for 5 minutes. This keeps the crispness and finishes cooking the birds. Or place in a microwave oven for 1 minute at baking power. Remove the birds from the skillet.

↳Serve the quail on a bed of steamed and seasoned Swiss chard and carrots.

↳Cooked rice, seasoned with parsley pesto, can be served as the grain for the meal.

↳Make a sauce by adding 1 cup of chicken stock or white wine to the skillet, stir in 2 tbs. Green Seasoning, or other prepared sauce, bring to a boil and reduce the liquid to ¼ cup, stir in 2 tsp. butter and serve immediately.

Linguine with Baby Clams

When you must have pasta, this dish is quick, easy and elegant. I use baby clams, which only need to be cooked for one or two minutes, any longer and they will be tough. Garlic and your favorite white wine give this dish its character. Use as much garlic as you can stand to make this sauce; although the guideline in the recipe is three cloves. The news is out, garlic is just plain good for you because it boosts immunity and protects against aging diseases. Clams will increase your calcium intake and help support the youthfulness in your bones. Even the parsley garnish is not to be missed, due to its protective vitamin C content.

Ingredients

4 oz. linguine pasta
3 garlic cloves, minced
½ onion, finely chopped
Sea salt or 2 anchovies crushed with red pepper flakes
5 large shiitake mushrooms, coarsely chopped
½ large red bell pepper, peeled, seeded and chopped
¼ cup white wine
1 tbs. spicy spaghetti seasoning mix
1 can whole baby clams
1 tbs. extra virgin olive oil
Chopped black olives for garnish
Chopped parsley for garnish

Steps

↔

↳Drain the clams using a colander and retain the juice.

↳ Heat a large skillet on medium high, add the olive oil, garlic and anchovies and stir until mixed. Then add onions and cook until they are soft.

↳ Add the peppers, mushrooms and seasoning, stir, reduce heat to low, cover and cook for 3-5 minutes until the mushrooms are done.

↳Uncover and add the wine and stir to prevent sticking. Add peppers and ¼ cup of the clam juice. Stir to mix and simmer for 2 or 3 minutes.

↳ Add baby clams, olives and parsley. Cook until heated, then remove from heat and keep warm.

↳Cook the linguine in a large pot of boiling salted water for 5-8 minutes, or according to the box instructions. When tender, drain and pour into a large bowl, top with the clam sauce and serve immediately.

↳Serve with a medley of steamed broccoli, zucchini and carrots.

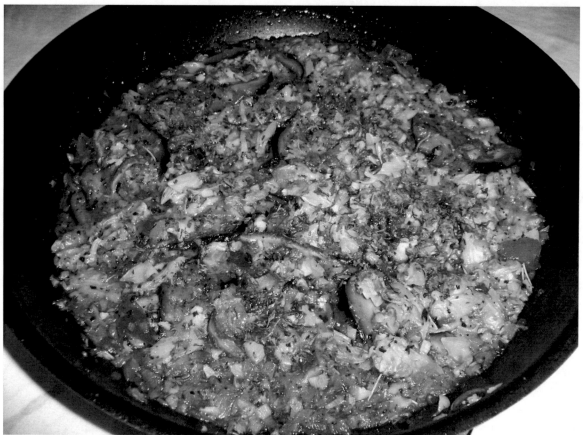

Figure 30 - Skillet ofLingume with Baby Clams

Baked Red Snapper

If you can get very fresh fish, this is your dish. You can remove the head or leave it as is. This is pure protein, naturally low-fat, quick and easy. Once you have the Green Seasoning (see contents) made you are ready to go. You owe it to your palate to make a batch of this powerful herb-flavored Green Seasoning

Ingredients

1 small whole red snapper
1 tsp. mild pepper sauce
2 tbs. Green Seasoning
1 tsp. salt
1 tsp. olive oil

Steps

↪Wash the fish well; remove any leftover scales, then make 3 large cuts through the skin of the fish with a sharp knife. Spoon the Green Seasoning over the fish and rub in well.

↪Sprinkle with salt and a dash of hot sauce.

↪Marinate for 10 to 20 minutes.

↪Place the fish in a greased baking dish. Cover with foil and bake in a preheated oven at 400 degrees F for 30 minutes until the fish is cooked and flakes easily when tested with a fork.

↪This fish can also be cooked in a microwave oven for 5-7 minutes.

↪Serve with the tomato sauce recipe (see pg. 173) on a bed of steamed kale, along with quinoa salad.

Cornish Hens

Make a change from chicken or turkey and choose Cornish hens. You will find them in the frozen section, along with turkey and other birds. They do not have as much fat as chicken, and you will not need to remove the skin. They are just perfect for entertaining a small group or celebrating your 'eat younger' attitude. These birds are on my menu almost every Christmas. For me, they are the epitome of celebration.

Ingredients

2 Cornish hens
2 tbs. extra virgin olive oil
2 large cloves garlic
1 tbs. each of finely chopped fresh thyme and rosemary
2 finely chopped green onions
2 tbs. soy sauce
Freshly ground black pepper and salt
For the peas and rice:
½ cup basmati rice
1 cup chicken stock or salted water
3 tbs. chopped parsley
½ cup frozen baby green peas
½ tbs. butter or ghee

Steps

↰—————————————————————————————————————→

↳Preheat oven to 450 degrees F.

↳Rub the hens with oil. Sprinkle some salt and pepper. Mix the garlic, thyme, rosemary and green onion together. Loosen the breast skin off each hen with your fingers, and then place some of the herbs mixture under the skin of each bird. Spread the remaining herbs over the bird and brush with soy sauce. Place the hens on a roasting rack. Transfer to a roasting pan. Add ¼ cup of water to the bottom of the pan.

↳Roast the hens for 15 minutes, baste the hens and reduce the oven temperature to 325 degrees F and continue cooking for another 15 to 20 minutes until the birds are well done. Juices run clear when pierced at the leg joints.

↳Retain the juices from the roasting pan. Cook the frozen peas for 1 minute in the juices in a microwave oven.

↳Add the half-cup of rice to the stock in a saucepan. Bring to a boil, reduce heat to low, cover and cook for 15 minutes. Stir in peas, parsley and butter.

↳Season with white pepper and serve with sautéed vegetables of your choice.

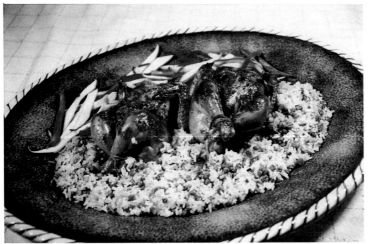

Figure 31 - Cornish Hens

Crab Burger

This is high quality, very simple food. When you really want a burger but your taste buds are not excited about ground beef, make it a crab burger! I got the idea for this when I was on vacation by the sea and a "claw burger" showed up as a choice in the burger section of the menu. It was exactly what I was wishing for at the time. If possible, use very fresh lump crabmeat and you will be delighted. The crab is naturally low in saturated fat, and the oil used in this recipe has the best smoke point for pan-frying the healthy way.

Ingredients

½ medium onion, finely chopped
½ medium finely chopped red sweet pepper
8 oz. lump crab meat
1 large egg
1 tsp. sweet relish
2 tsp. mayonnaise
3 tbs. grape seed oil
1 garlic clove, minced
½ cup breadcrumbs seasoned with ½ tsp. dried thyme
½ tsp. salt and pepper to taste

Steps

↩In a medium hot skillet, sauté the garlic clove in 1 tablespoon of the oil. Add the onion, red pepper, salt and pepper to the pan and cook until soft. Remove from skillet and let cool.

↩Meanwhile, thoroughly press all excess moisture from the crabmeat using a colander or strainer.

↩In a medium bowl, combine the onion mixture with the crabmeat. Add ¼ cup of seasoned breadcrumbs, the beaten egg, relish mayonnaise and a dash of salt and pepper.

↩Form 4 medium patties and squeeze any excess liquid from the patties as you shape them. Place the remaining breadcrumbs in a shallow dish and lightly press the patties into the breadcrumbs, coating each side, then dust off excess breadcrumbs, place patties on a plate and chill in the refrigerator for 30 minutes.

↩Pan fry patties on medium heat, in 2 tbs. of grape seed oil until they are brown on both sides, about 3 minutes per side.

↩Serve with sautéed white cabbage and thinly sliced red peppers, seasoned with a dash of white balsamic vinegar, salt and pepper on whole-wheat buns.

↩ Serves 2.

Grilled Salmon Steaks with Orange Sauce

Salmon has omega-3 oil, which is a great fat. It helps to lubricate your skin, and keep it looking younger. You will notice that there is no need to add fat or oil to this fish. The fish has just the right amount of natural oil to get it through the short cooking process. Your heart will jump for joy if you eat fish at least twice per week. Eating this way will help to balance your cholesterol, keep your blood vessels healthy and increase your zest and vitality. This is a quick recipe that will make you happier and take your dining soul to a higher level. The sauce for this recipe is made with shallots. Shallots are in the onion family but are smaller than onions and have a coppery brown or pinkish skin. They have an onion-garlicky flavor that lends a tasty complexity to sauces.

Ingredients

2 salmon steaks about 4-5 oz. each
½ tsp. dill weed
1 tsp. onion powder
½ lemon, squeezed
1 tsp. olive oil
Sea salt and freshly ground pepper
Sauce for steaks
½ cup fish stock or dry white wine
Juice of one orange
1 tbs. of orange zest (peel zest from the orange with a citrus zester or sharp knife)
2 shallots
1 clove garlic, minced
1 tbs. clarified butter or ghee (recipe in this book pg. 172)
2 tsp. canola oil
Pinch of salt and pepper

Steps

↶Squeeze the lemon over the salmon and sprinkle on the dill, onion powder, salt and pepper.

↶Set aside for 15 minutes to marinate.

↶Meanwhile, pre-heat your grill to high, then reduce to medium high.

↶Brush your grill with oil to prevent the fish from sticking, and place steaks on grill and cook 5 minutes without moving. Turn and grill other side for about 3 minutes or until the fish is cooked through.

↶Adjust salt and pepper

↶Serve with a hearty quinoa salad in salad section of this book, steamed carrots and snow peas, and garnish with orange wedges.

Sauce: Sauté garlic and shallots in canola oil for 2 minutes, add the stock or wine and the orange juice and zest. Simmer until the sauce is reduced by half and begins to thicken. Add the butter, salt and pepper. Stir and remove from the heat. Serve immediately over the salmon.

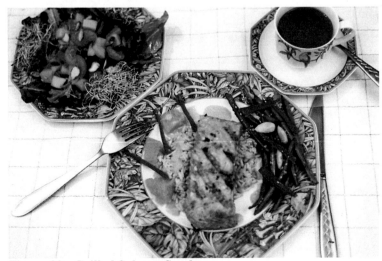

Figure 32 - Grilled Salmon Steaks

Potato Frittata

For those days when you just feel like cooking an omelet, make an upscale version by adding potatoes and peppers, and there you have it, a dinner frittata. Serve this with a hefty green salad and homemade dressing and you will have a very fortifying meal. Eggs are experiencing a revival in the food realm since the link to high cholesterol is diminishing with continuing evidence of the complications of that syndrome. Eggs are high in B vitamins, which help keep energy high. They contain lutein, an antioxidant that helps to keep eyes healthy and to protect your cardiovascular system. So, this meal is actually high in some of the essentials that keep your body slowing the aging process.

Ingredients

3 medium red potatoes, peeled and thinly sliced, horizontally
2 tsp. olive oil
½ medium onion, thinly sliced
1 large garlic clove, minced
½ red bell pepper, thinly sliced
½ yellow bell pepper, thinly sliced
1 large jalapeno pepper, seeded and minced
2 oz. smoked pork chop, finely diced (optional)
¼ cup fresh Italian parsley or cilantro
2 egg whites and 1 whole large egg (use 3 eggs if you want the lecithin from the yolks for better brain function)
Salt and pepper to taste and Bleu cheese crumbles for garnish

Steps

↰Rinse the potato slices in cold water and dry. Sprinkle with salt.

↰Heat the oil in a large non-stick skillet over medium heat. Spread the potato slices evenly in the skillet and cook over moderate heat. Turn when brown and cook the other side until the potatoes are cooked.

↰Add the onion, garlic and pepper. Cook on low heat, stirring until soft for about 3 minutes.

↰Preheat the broiler.

↰Add the finely diced pork chop and parsley to the pot and cook stirring about 1 minute.

↰Beat the egg and egg whites and add to the skillet. Cook until eggs are set. Remove skillet to oven broiler. Add cheese crumbles.

↰Cook eggs on top by placing them under the broiler until brown, about 1 minute.

Slice frittata and serve with sweet red pepper sauce recipe in this book.

Sea Scallops

Fresh sea scallops are such pure food. I think that the only way they should be eaten is raw, topped with a great lime marinade. Because we can't always have the luxury of freshness, the scallops in this recipe are pan seared after being marinated with our Green Seasoning and served with a butternut squash cream sauce. This adds the excitement of color to the dish. Serve with a green salad mix and dressing from this book. This recipe gets you out of the kitchen fast. This is almost effortless, because the squash is cooked in the microwave oven, and scallops naturally cook in 2-3 minutes. This is low fat and high in protein, with the delicate balance of a high nutrient carbohydrate like butternut squash.

Ingredients

1 small butternut squash
1 cup of fish stock or 1 bouillon cube dissolved in one cup of water
¼ large onion
2 tbs. cream
¼ tsp. grated nutmeg
8 fresh sea scallops
1 tsp. salt and fresh ground black pepper
1 tbs. Green Seasoning - see recipe in sauces section
1 tbs. grape seed oil and 1 tsp. ghee

Steps

➔Bake butternut squash in microwave for 8 to 10 minutes. Cool, cut in half and scoop out 1 cup.

➔Place squash, onion, ½ cup of stock, and spice in a high-powered blender and blend until smooth. Add more stock if the mixture is too thick, until you get the consistency you desire in a sauce. Add the cream and stir.

➔Add salt, pepper and the Green Seasoning to the scallops and let marinate for 5 minutes. To cook the scallops, place a non-stick skillet over moderate high heat until hot. Add the ghee and oil to the skillet, then add the scallops and cook until brown on one side, about 2-3 minutes. Turn and brown on the other side about 1 ½-2 minutes.

➔To serve, spread the butternut sauce on the bottom of a plate then place a ¼ cup of the grain of your choice and top with the 4 scallops. This goes well with grains like cooked quinoa or rice.

➔Add a salad of your choice from this book to add more vegetables to this menu.

➔Serves 2.

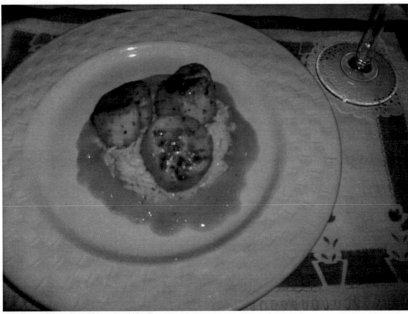

Figure 33 - Scallops with Butternut cream sauce

Shepherds Pie

The potato makes this dish very comforting. The beauty of this recipe is that along with comfort you take in a whole lot of age-fighting, stamina-building vegetables like shiitake mushrooms, soymilk and carrots. This is a complete meal giving you protein, carbohydrates and fat, in reasonable balance. This recipe makes 2 servings.

Ingredients

½ lb. ground lamb
1 tsp. olive oil
½ bell pepper, peeled and chopped
1 carrot, peeled and finely diced
½ large onion, finely chopped
1 fresh tomato, pureed
5 large shiitake mushrooms, finely chopped
1 tbs. bouquet garni or 1 tsp. thyme, 5 peppercorns, ½-tsp. rosemary and a bay leaf, all dried
1 large potato, baked in the microwave for 10 minutes, cooled and grated
1 egg
½ cup milk
½ cup beef stock (or use a beef stock cube)
White cheddar cheese, grated
Salt and pepper or hot sauce to taste

Steps

↳Season the ground lamb with salt and pepper and brown over medium heat in a large non-stick skillet.

↳Add the oil, vegetables and herbs and cook stirring until the vegetables are cooked. Add stock, a little at a time, as the vegetables are cooking to prevent it from getting too dry.

↳Whisk the egg with milk and mix with the grated potatoes.

↳Place the meat and vegetable mixture in a greased baking pie dish.

↳Spread the potato mixture on top.

↳Bake 20 minutes at 350 degrees F.

↳Serve with a baby greens salad and a dressing from this book.

Shrimp Curry

There is no other spice like curry. It is so tantalizing and there are many regional versions of Indian curry. I have always known of curry; it is a well-established street food in my birthplace, Trinidad. Trinidad's curry powder is becoming known as one of the best blends available in America by celebrity chefs. Curry powder will lose its flavor very quickly, so buy the powder in grocery stores that sell spices from bins, since they tend to be more flavorful. The spices of curry are said to have properties that relieve aches and pains associated with aging. Curries sometimes have coconut milk. Coconut milk is usually sold in cans in the section of the grocery store with Asian food. Do not use sweetened coconut milk.

Ingredients

½ pound peeled, de-veined shrimp seasoned with 1 tbs. lime juice and salt
2 small white skin potatoes, coarsely chopped into 1-inch cubes
1 carrot, coarsely chopped
1 medium eggplant, cut into ½-inch cubes
1 large onion, finely chopped
1 small (about 1-inch) piece of fresh ginger, peeled and finely chopped
2 garlic pods
1 tsp. each cumin and coriander seeds, toasted and ground
2 pods cardamom, toasted and smashed to get the full flavor of the seeds
1 tbs. curry powder
1 tbs. canola oil, plus 1 tsp. ghee or butter
1 ½ cups of fish stock or salted water
½ cup unsweetened coconut milk
2 tsp. Pickapeppa sauce, available in most grocery stores
¼ cup cilantro
½ tsp salt, black pepper and hot sauce to your taste

Steps

←——————————————————————————→

↳Place canola oil and 1 peeled and crushed garlic pod in a large heavy bottom skillet and heat over medium heat until garlic is light brown. After flavor is released, remove pod from pot and discard.

↳Add onion, 1 minced garlic pod, ginger, ground cumin, coriander and cardamom to the skillet and stir-fry until tender. Pour ¼ cup of water or stock in a small bowl, add the curry powder and stir until mixed. Add the mixture to the skillet and cook for 2-3 minutes.

↳Add potatoes, carrots, water or stock and coconut milk, cook for 10 minutes.

↳Then add the rest of the vegetables and small amounts of water, if the sauce is too thick. Cook on low heat until all vegetables are tender. Roll the cilantro leaves and snip with a kitchen scissors.

↳Add the Pickapeppa sauce, hot sauce, and adjust the salt, garnish with minced cilantro.

↳Add the seasoned shrimp and ghee and simmer for 2-3 minutes until shrimp is pink.

↳Serve with basmati rice and green salad of your choice.

Grilled Mahi Mahi with Curry Sauce

Mahi Mahi is a meaty firm fish. It is excellent for grilling. This is served with a curry sauce, which will make your heart youthful. Fish is a good way to pack in protein without overloading on saturated fat. Proteins provide amino acids that help to make necessary enzymes that speed up all the processes in your cells, keep your heart operating at optimum levels, and you from gaining weight. The fat in this recipe is ghee, also known as clarified butter or a de-hydrogenated body friendly fat. This recipe has ancient East Indian origins, hence the use of ghee. It gives the curry a great flavor even when used in small amounts. And research has shown that we need about 10% saturated fat per day.

Ingredients

2 small mahi mahi steaks, each weighing about 6 oz.
Juice of ½ lime
¼ cup plain low fat yogurt
1 tsp. curry powder
Dash of salt and pepper
Ingredients for sauce
2 tsp. ghee plus 2 tsp. canola oil
2 garlic cloves, one crushed and one whole
½ small onion, finely chopped
½ tsp. ground cumin
2 tsp. curry powder
½ tsp. dried thyme or leaves from 3 sprigs of fresh thyme
½ cup of semi-dry white wine
½ tsp. salt and ¼ tsp. hot pepper sauce

Steps

↪Wash and pat dry the fish, season with salt and pepper.

↪Mix the lime juice with the yogurt and coat both sides of the fish. Spread the curry powder over both sides of the fish and set aside in the refrigerator for ½ hour or longer.

↪Put the canola oil in a ridged grill pan or heavy iron skillet over high heat.

↪Add the fish and cook 4 to 5 five minutes without turning. After 4 minutes check to see if the grill marks are brown but not black. Turn fish and cook about 3 minutes. Keep warm.

↪Prepare the sauce; in a saucepan sauté one garlic pod in the oil mixture until it is brown but not burnt. Remove and discard pod. Add crushed garlic, onion, cumin and thyme. Cook by stir-frying over medium heat until onions are translucent, about 3 -5 minutes. Stir the curry powder into a small amount of water, mix well and then stir into the mixture in the saucepan. Add white wine, salt and hot sauce and simmer for about 10 minutes until the mixture is reduced by half. Pour sauce in a blender and puree. Strain and pour into a small saucepan. Add the ghee or butter; warm over low heat to mix in the butter. Taste and adjust the seasoning. Pour sauce on the bottom of your plate. Place fish on top of sauce. Surround with steamed vegetables, such as carrots, yellow squash, green peas and green beans. Serve with basmati rice.

↪Serves two.

↪Enjoy.

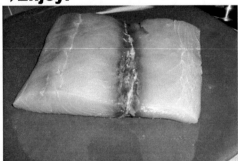

Figure 34 - Fresh Mahi Mahi Fillet

Rosemary Roast Chicken

Let your inner chef come out and really play with this bird. Cooking a bird for one person might seem like too much, but it is a real budget saver, and that's a beautiful thing. The meat can be used for two or three meals. Part of the breast can be reserved for a curried chicken salad, or a Mexican wrap with goat cheese and assorted peppers. The legs and thighs of the bird can be separated and eaten with vegetables and grains for a main meal, and the remains of the bird can be used in your favorite chicken soup recipe.

Ingredients

One large fresh chicken, rubbed with fresh lime, rinsed and patted dry
4 sprigs of fresh rosemary or 1-2 tbs. dried rosemary
1 tbs. olive oil
2 tbs. soy sauce for basting
½ cup of your favorite white wine
Salt and coarsely ground pepper

Steps

↩Preheat the oven to 425 degrees F.

↩Loosen the breast skin with your fingers and place a sprig of rosemary under the skin on each side of the breast. Put some rosemary in the cavity of the bird. Rub the olive oil all over the bird, then sprinkle with pepper and brush all over with the soy sauce.

↩Place the chicken, breast side up, on the rack of a roasting pan.

↩Add wine to the bottom of the pan and place a sprig of rosemary in the water.

↩Roast for 20 minutes at 425 degrees F. Baste, lower the heat to 350 degrees F and continue roasting for 45-50 minutes until the bird is a beautiful brown and the juices run clear when pierced with a fork in the leg joint. If using a thermometer, the internal temperature should be 165-170 degrees F.

↩Transfer the chicken to a platter and let rest for 15 minutes before carving.

↩Pour the juices from the roasting pan into a saucepan. Add one minced shallot, a dash of salt and pepper and heat until reduced by half and the shallots are cooked. Remove the chicken fat from the gravy by using a beaker with a fat separator, or cool the gravy and remove the hardened fat from the top.

To enrich the de-fatted sauce, warm and add one tablespoon of cream or butter to the sauce.

Sauces, Seasonings and Marinades

Sauces add flavor or intensify flavor in food preparation. They also enhance moisture and can add color to the plate when presenting the food. Seasonings can be used to give distinctive character to a dish and help to build specific flavors of regional foods.

But that's not all. For instance, turmeric, the ingredient that gives curry powders its distinctive orange-yellow color, also has curcumin, which has an anti-inflammatory effect on the body. Just by adding curry to your diet, you can help slow your aging, feel great and never experience a host of aging problems, including arthritis and irritable bowel syndrome. There are two recipes with curry sauce in the dinner section of this book. However, be aware of sauces that add an overload of sugar and saturated fat. Usually this is the case with store-bought bottled sauces. It is wise to read labels of commercial sauces to make sure that you are not unaware of increasing your sugar, or glycemic load.

Marinades are usually made of wine, vinegar, citrus juices, oil and other herbs or spices, with the purpose of making fish and meat more tender and flavorful.

Ghee

Prepare the ghee by placing 8 ounces of unsalted butter in a small saucepan. Heat on very low temperature until all the solids in the butter settle at the bottom of the pan, about 20 minutes. Do not let the butter boil; just simmer. Froth will form on the surface. As the heating continues, it will disappear and the milk solids will fall to the bottom.
It takes just a short while to develop a tremendous amount of buttery flavor. When the solids are on the bottom and the liquid butter is clear, strain through cheesecloth into a small glass jar.

When using recipes that contain butter, you can use less ghee than butter and get a real explosive butter flavor. You can also buy ghee at middle-eastern and specialty food grocery stores. The "eat younger" benefit of this is that you not only get intensified buttery flavor, but the process helps to lessen the effects of saturated fat on the cardiovascular system.

Tomato Sauce for Fish

Use this sauce on grilled and pan-fried fish. I taught one of my cousins how to make this sauce and I was amazed at his creativity in finding things on which to use it. He put it on eggs, chicken breasts, pasta and roasted vegetables. I was also impressed with how long it kept in the refrigerator. I learned this in a cooking class with a chef in Puerto Vallarta, Mexico. He used Serrano peppers. I use jalapeno peppers because I have a ton of them in my garden and my cousin used a commercial Scotch Bonnet pepper sauce. So let your creative sauces flow and have a wild time with this sauce.

Ingredients

6 Roma or plum tomatoes
1 tbs. olive oil and 1 tsp. butter
1 Jalapeno pepper, seeded and finely chopped
1 bay leaf
2 tbs. chopped cilantro
1 tsp. white pepper
½ small white onion or shallots finely chopped
2 crushed and finely chopped garlic cloves
1 tbs. fresh oregano leaves, finely chopped
¼ cup white wine
1 tsp. sea salt

Steps

← ———————————————————————————————— →

✍ **Make a cross cut at the tips of the tomatoes and plunge them into boiling water for 1 minute. Remove from water and immediately place in a bowl of ice-cold water. When the tomatoes are cooled, peel off the skin, starting at the cross cut and coarsely chop them and set aside. Sauté onion, garlic and pepper in 1 tbs. oil over medium high heat until they begin to soften. Add oregano, salt and white pepper and continue to sauté, lowering heat to medium. Add tomatoes and continue to cook. Finally, add wine, bay leaf, salt and pepper, lower heat and continue to cook for 5 minutes.**
✍ **Cool sauce, remove bay leaf and place in blender with 1 tsp. of butter and blend well.**
✍ **Serve on grilled fish or whatever else your imagination leads you to.**

Green Seasoning

This is a traditional Trinidadian seasoning that can be used to season meat, fish or chicken. It can be made in single batches or can be made in bulk and stored in the fridge. It is also sold commercially in grocery stores in the Caribbean. Green seasoning is used in some of the recipes in this book. The small sweet pimento peppers in the Caribbean have a special distinct flavor that gives this seasoning its distinguishable taste.

Ingredients

Pods from 2 bulbs of garlic
1 bunch of green onions
3 pimento peppers or ½ green bell pepper and ½ red bell pepper
1 hot scotch bonnet pepper or hot pepper sauce to taste (optional)
3 stalks of celery
1 bunch fresh thyme about 5 sprigs, use leaves only
½ bunch parsley, stems discarded
¼ cup of shadon beni or cilantro leaves
2 inches of fresh ginger
¼ cup fresh squeezed lime juice

Steps

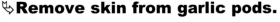

↳ Remove skin from garlic pods.
↳ Place all other ingredients in a blender and process until well mixed.
↳ Put blended seasoning in a glass jar and store in the refrigerator.
↳ Use to season any meat for a real West Indian taste.

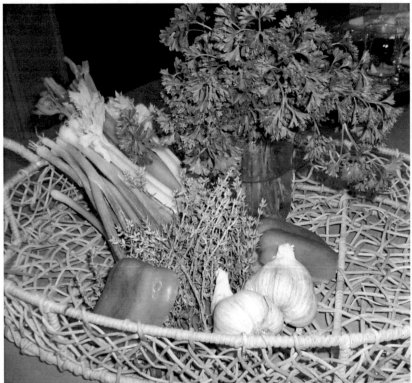

Figure 35 - Fresh ingredients for Green Seasoning

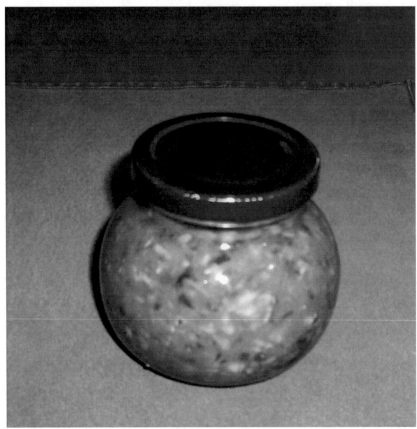

Figure 36 - Freahly made Green Seasoning

Sweet Red Pepper Sauce

This red pepper sauce is a great improvement on gravy. It is chock-full of the right stuff, like vitamins A and E and bioflavonoids to scare away your free radicals from disrupting cell and organ function. Red peppers are also high in vitamin C, which promotes the formation of collagen, which makes your skin beautiful. Use it every chance you get. It is a great way to get some of your "5 a day" vegetables. And it tastes good. If you like your sauce spicy you can make this as fiery as you like.

Ingredients

1 tsp. butter plus 2 tsp. grape seed oil
½ medium onion, finely chopped
1 plum tomato, seeded and diced
½ tsp. Pickapeppa Sauce
¼ cup non-fat plain yogurt
2 garlic cloves
2 sweet red peppers, peeled and seeded
1 tsp. ground white pepper
2 bay leaves
1 cup chicken broth or salted water
Salt and pepper to taste

Steps

↜Use a large skillet to sauté garlic in oil, over medium heat until soft.

↜Add onions and peppers and sauté for 2 minutes.

↜Add tomatoes, bay leaves, Pickapeppa sauce and white pepper to saucepan, stirring well to break up the tomatoes. Add water or chicken broth and simmer for 10 minutes. ↜Remove bay leaves.

↜Place ingredients in a blender and blend until smooth.

↜Adjust the taste for salt and pepper.

↜Add yogurt and butter and serve over your favorite meat or chicken.

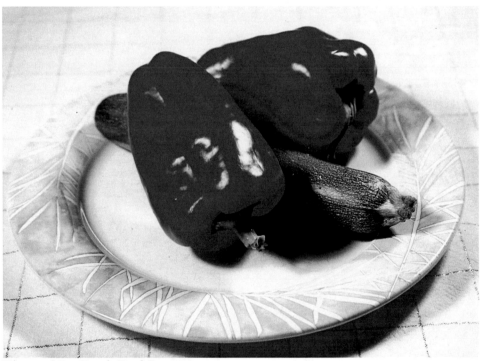

Figure 37 - Fresh Red Peppers

Apple Dill and Rosemary Sauce

Use this sauce when you are feeling festive. The apple, dill and rosemary combine to give you an herby sweetness that delights the palate. This recipe uses fresh mustard seeds. These seeds have natural anti-cancer properties and the ability to decrease the production of inflammation. This can bring relief to symptoms of asthma and rheumatoid arthritis. I have used fresh pureed apples or a jar of organic, no-sugar-added baby apple sauce to make this recipe; either way you get great apple flavor.

Ingredients

2 tsp. grape seed oil plus 2 tsp. ghee
1 tsp. mustard seeds
1 large shallot, finely diced
1 tsp. dried rosemary
1 tsp. dried dill weed
1 large shallot
½ cup Vermouth or white wine
1 jar of organic baby apple sauce
1 tsp. honey
½ cup chicken stock
Dash of salt and pepper or hot sauce

Steps

↳Heat the oil and ghee in a medium skillet over medium high heat.

↳Add mustard seeds and cover skillet until you hear them stop popping, about 1minute.

↳Add chopped shallots, rosemary and dill and cook until the shallots are soft and the herbs give up their flavor, about 2-3 minutes.

↳Add white wine, apple sauce, and the chicken stock and cook until the sauce is reduced by half. Season with salt and pepper, and for sweetness add the honey.

↳Use with grilled salmon or pork tenderloin. This sauce will keep in the fridge for up to 2 weeks.

Avocado Sauce

Avocadoes are so wonderful, with their marvelous slow aging properties like brain support and essential fats, that you should grasp every opportunity to use them.
Here is a creamy, sophisticated sauce that you can make in a jiffy to give lean fish and chicken breasts a gourmet appearance.

Ingredients

1 California avocado
1 tbs. apple cider vinegar, white balsamic vinegar or fresh lime juice
2 green onions
1 anchovy fillet
1 small jalapeno pepper, seeded
2 tbs. chopped cilantro
1 tbs. olive oil

Steps

⮑Place all ingredients in a food processor and blend until smooth.
⮑Place fish on plate.
⮑Serve over fish.
⮑Enjoy!

Marinade for Fish

If you always wanted to cook fish but are in a quandary about how to start, just go with this marinade. Fish will pick up the flavor of a marinade in 15-20 minutes. Anything more is overkill. You can change the herbs in your marinade to add the distinctive flavor that you desire.

Ingredients

1 tbs. white balsamic vinegar
1 tsp. juice of fresh lime
1 tsp. sea salt
½ tsp. freshly grated black pepper
3 tbs. fresh cilantro leaves, minced
2 tbs. canola or extra virgin olive oil

Steps

⟷

↳In a bowl mix all ingredients, except the oil.

↳Slowly whisk in the oil until well mixed.

↳Pour over the fish and let stand for 20 minutes in the fridge.

↳Cook fish as desired.

Glossary

Acid: Any of a class of chemical compounds that are characterized by low pH (hydrogen ion concentration). A pH scale measures the relative acidity or alkalinity of substances. The scale runs from 0 to 14. A pH of 7 is considered neutral. Numbers below 7 denote increasing acidity and numbers above 7 denote increasing alkalinity. Stomach acid, coffee and coco cola have pH between 2 and 3. Blood and water are close to 7 and soap is alkaline with ph between 10 and 13.

Amino acid: Any of twenty-two nitrogen containing organic acids, which are the chemical building blocks of proteins. Some amino acids are considered essential; a term used for nutrients needed for building and repair that cannot be made by the body, and therefore must be eaten as part of the diet. Essential amino acids are found in animal products that include lean meats, fish, poultry, milk, yogurt, cheese and eggs.

Antioxidant:. A substance that blocks or inhibits destructive oxidative reactions in the body. These reactions occur in the body most often when oxygen reacts with another substance, resulting in free radicals. Free radicals are unpaired oxygen atoms that occur because of metabolism and oxidative stress. They have at least one unpaired electron and are highly reactive. They can cause damage to cells. Scientific investigators think that free radicals play a role in the development of cancer, heart disease and the natural process of aging. The most popular antioxidants are beta-carotene, vitamin C, vitamin E and selenium. They are found in plants such as fruits, vegetables and nuts.

Bioflavonoid: Any of a group of biologically active plant substances called flavonoids. They are essential for the stability and absorption of vitamin C into the body. They are not vitamins, but are sometimes referred to as vitamin P.

Collagen: The fibrous protein found in bone, cartilage, and connective tissues of the body.

Chinese Five-Spice Powder: The classic five spices that make up this powder are star anise, Szechwan pepper, fennel, cloves and cinnamon. It is available at most supermarkets and Asian food stores.

Enzyme: One of many specific proteins produced by all living organisms. Its function is to start or speed up chemical reactions without being consumed.

Folate: Associated with Folic Acid, a member of the B-complex vitamins. It is essential for the growth and repair of tissue and the formation of red blood cells. It is found in lentils, chickpeas, green leafy vegetables, fresh fruit, liver and yeast. The daily requirement for healthy people is 400 micrograms (mcg).

Garam Masala: A dry-roasted mixture of ground spices used in East Indian cooking and sold in East Indian markets. Garam is the Indian word for "hot" and masala means "spices." It is an aromatic blend and might contain combinations of black pepper, cumin, cinnamon, cardamom, cloves, mace, nutmeg, and coriander and can add a pleasant flavor to soups, sauces and curries.

Honing Steel: A tool for sharpening knives. It is usually sold in stores that sell professional kitchen knives. It helps to realign the edge of the blade and keep it sharp.
It should be used frequently, if not every time you use your blade. The instrument has a handle with a guard and a long shaft of steel. To sharpen your knife, hold the steel by the handle with the shaft vertically upright. With the knife in the opposite hand, starting with the tip of the blade, pull the blade down the shaft at a 22 degree angle. Repeat on each side of the blade about 4 or 5 times

Immune System: A complex system in the body that depends on the interaction of many different organs, cells and diet. It's function is to identify and destroy harmful foreign substances like viruses and bacteria. It also has to identify your own cells as part of the many systems it oversees and not attack or destroy them.

Metabolism: The physical and chemical processes necessary to maintain life. It involves the production of cellular energy by breaking down the food we eat and making biological substances to maintain life.

Phytochemical: Any one of many substances present in fruits and vegetables that have various health-promoting characteristics. Some phytochemicals appear to have protective properties for the body.

Saturated Fat: A chemical compound that has fatty acid molecules as part of its structure. The fatty acid is said to be saturated if it contains as many hydrogen atoms as its structure will allow. Fat molecules with fatty acids that can incorporate one additional hydrogen atom is said to be monounsaturated, and those that can incorporate two or more hydrogen atoms are said to be polyunsaturated. The human body demands a delicate balance of these molecules to maintain excellent health.

Index

R

raspberries, 45
red snapper, 152
ritual, 38, 39, 40
Rituals, 12
Roast chicken, 169

S

salmon, 10, 23, 28, 30, 34, 35, 67, 71, 75, 103, 157, 158
Salmon Steaks, 157
salsa, 33, 34, 35, 47, 79
Salted Cod, 58
Sardines, 23, 28, 59
Saturated Fat, 185
sea scallops, 161
Sea scallops, 31
Sesame Seed, 117
shiitake mushrooms, 35, 54, 141, 142, 149, 163
Smoothie, 24
snacks, 4
Soups, 81, 82
soymilk, 20, 24
spinach, 33, 75, 87, 137, 138, 144, 145
Split pea soup, 99
starchy carbohydrate, 10, 57, 99, 145
strawberries, 24, 29, 31, 36, 41, 60, 80, 137, 138
Strawberry spinach salad, 33
Sweet Red Pepper Sauce, 177
Sword Fish, 28

T

tabbouleh, 140
tabouli, 34, 111, 139, 140

Tabouli, 24, 29
Taro or dasheen leaves, 87
tea, 20, 23, 24, 28, 29, 30, 31, 33, 34, 35, 36, 57, 63, 64
Toasted sesame oil, 111
Tomato coconut soup, 36
tomato sauce, 28
Tools, 8
Traditions, 12

U

U.S. Department of Agriculture (USDA), 145

V

Vegetable stock, 107
vitamin C, 59, 60, 75, 139
vitamin E, 41, 43, 62, 110

W

wheat germ, 41, 42, 44
white balsamic, 111, 113, 114, 117, 118, 135, 137, 144, 182
whole grain bread, 18

Y

yogurt, 29, 36, 37, 44, 45, 49, 50, 53, 60, 112, 114, 121, 122, 124, 167, 168, 177, 178, 183
younger, 15
youthfulness, 14

Z

zest, 14, 103, 113, 117, 127, 157, 158
zinc, 131